Wes Cole's Healthy Habits

Wes Cole's

Healthy Habits

How to Change Your
Diet and Exercise Habits
for Lifelong Fitness

Wes Cole

McBooks Press
Ithaca, New York

Published by McBooks Press 2012

Copyright © 2012 by Wes Cole

Cover photo of Wes and Beth Cole by Machelle Moody of Mac's Photography ©2011.
Dust jacket and interior design by Panda Musgrove.

Library of Congress Cataloging-in-Publication Data

Cole, Wes, 1980-
 Wes Cole's healthy habits : how to change your diet and exercise habits for lifelong fitness / Wes Cole.
    p. cm.
 Summary: "This wellness guide presents a solution for taking control of diet and fitness. The detailed plan is broken down into four cycles, providing supportive guidance for gradually altering eating habits and eliminating harmful substances that promote weight gain. An active lifestyle is encouraged through realistic suggestions, until daily fitness becomes second nature. Formulating a patient and supportive approach to health, this handbook outlines a lifelong transformation, one step at a time"-- Provided by publisher.
 ISBN 978-1-59013-627-0 (pbk.)
 1. Physical fitness. 2. Exercise. 3. Nutrition. 4. Health. I. Title.
 RA781.C55 2012
 613--dc23

                         2012001551

Visit the McBooks Press website at www.mcbooks.com.

Printed in the United States of America
9 8 7 6 5 4 3 2 1

I dedicate this book to Beth
My love . . . my wife . . . my everything!
"We did it, baby!"

Contents

Part Two—The Four Cycles

Acknowledgments

For those who haven't yet read my author bio, I'm a long way from L.A. or New York, and I believe it's quite a feat that my program has made the noise it has considering that this whole thing started in a modest, 1500-square-foot gym in Tulsa, Oklahoma—not the first place that comes to mind when you think of fitness revolutions. As much as my ego wants me to believe it was purely my dynamic charisma, intelligence, and talent that brought this book into your hands today, unfortunately (or fortunately), there's more to the story. The reality is that writing and finding a way to have this book published has been one of the most challenging things I have ever done. In fact, it would have been impossible had it not been for a few special people, and I think I would be in serious trouble if I didn't mention them.

First, I thank my literary agent, Krista Goering. Before her, my experience with literary agents reminded me of dating a popular girl in high school: they were quick to lose interest in me, they really didn't care and, worst of all, they acted like they were doing me an epic favor by talking to me. Krista changed that for me, and her faith in my book and her kindness were a breath of fresh air.

I thank McBooks Press, my publisher, for caring more about the actual words in the book than the author's fame or platform. If it weren't for publishers like this, I'm afraid all books would be written by Paris Hilton and Britney Spears.

Despite this, *some* platform is necessary, and the man primarily responsible for the thimble-sized amount of fame and exposure that I have is Paul James (aka The Gardener Guy). Paul was a successful Healthy Habit Plan follower who paid, like everyone else, for my services. He owed me no favors yet for some reason he decided to help me break into TV, and that's when my career was put into hyperdrive. Thank you!

We all have dreams and although it's good to look to the horizon and have goals, in the meantime we all still have to make a living. A guy named Steve Cleveland helped me immeasurably in this regard. Steve pulled me off of a used car lot—(Yeah, I tried to sell cars for about a week, unsuccessfully!)—after I'd lost my job at a gym because I refused to push their protein shakes. Steve, a good friend, pulled me up out of total obscurity when no one, and I mean NO ONE, thought I was worth a sideways glance. To this day, I don't know exactly why you did it, Steve, but it's something I will always remember.

I want to mention my brother, Kyle. He was one of my most successful clients but he is also reassuring proof to me that there are people out there who are weirder than me. Underneath all that weirdness though is a great "kid" and a person who has the uncanny ability to make me laugh harder than anyone else I know.

I thank my father. He raised me with a firm hand and introduced me not only to the life-changing effects of martial arts but also taught me to believe that I could channel my immense energy to do great things. This was important, considering that I acted like a little Tasmanian devil as a child. If it weren't for my father, I think my only claim to fame would be an appearance on *America's Most Wanted*.

I thank my mother who is the type of person who would risk life and limb and get out of her car on the highway to rescue an injured pigeon. I was always a little different, and my mother was the type of person who saw it only as uniqueness and taught me to do the same.

Thanks as well to my Grandma Sears who passed away during the spring of 2010. She was an exceptional woman whose life story could easily be a best seller (maybe my next book), although she would come back and haunt me if I didn't donate every penny made from that life story of hers to a church or charity, because that was her legacy. She was the epitome of selflessness, and I believe people like her go straight to Heaven on the express lane.

Thanks to my Grandma Jones, who taught me the importance of an education and gifted me the ability to read anything. Once I started, I never stopped, and I can't think of anything in this world that would make her happier than reading her grandson's very own book. Her incredible faith, honesty, and goodness are guideposts that I will strive to match each and every day of my life, but it is something I will certainly fall short of.

Thank you to my Grandpa Jones, who has passed away as well but was a real-life genius. If I do someday come up with any brilliant ideas, I'll owe it to his genes. I love you, Grandpa, and I miss your strong farmer's hugs.

Thank you to all the real martial artists out there who still crawl off their cozy couches and continue to train. It was in this type of environment I learned that excellence was not a chore but a habit.

In my life, there have been a few individuals who seemed to have been put into the world to sidetrack me, scare me, and try, with all their hearts, to put pessimistic thoughts into my head. I once wondered why these people existed but now I know. I also dedicate this book to all of those who didn't believe in me. Your negativity drove me more than you'll ever know. You all know who you are . . . and so do I.

Love and thanks to my son, Jax, who has shown me that there is a level of love that I never before knew existed.

And last but not least, I thank a special woman of mine, my wife, Beth; a woman who not only tirelessly believed in me and *Wes Cole's*

Healthy Habits but also was an instrumental part of the research, development, and editing of this book. She is a woman who watched my big dreams immensely stress our relationship for years, but who persevered out of pure blind faith in me and my abilities. She is much more than just a great, supportive partner. For a long time before I met her, people always used to ask me, "Wes, when are you going to get a life?" She gave me that life, and I count my blessings each and every day that she was put *into* my life.

Preface

So you diet and diet.

You've cleared out your kitchen and married your treadmill.

You've confronted your emotional eating and you know all about the fat cell.

You're headlong into low-carb, high-fiber, and fat-free everything.

The perfect recipe for permanent weight loss, right?

So, where's your fairy-tale ending?

Why aren't you one of those before and after pictures in the magazines?

"Results Not Typical." Oh, yeah. That's the truth.

Diet books and fitness gurus would have you believe that it's all about your motivation, your drive, your willpower, and your discipline—or your lack thereof.

So, there you are. Suddenly, some personal character flaw high-lighted and blamed for your failure, as if you didn't already feel bad enough. But you're obviously not alone. Obesity is an epidemic. Could those fitness gurus be right? Are we Americans—*an entire country*—really that lazy or undisciplined, utterly incapable of traveling the well-researched path to health?

There's more to the story.

What diet books forget to tell you is that the "path to health" leads straight into a dense forest and right up a mountain, probably a volcano. They don't tell you, and so you don't show up prepared. It's like the first day of kindergarten and no one told you to bring your crayons.

Failure is not entirely your fault. Sure, you carry some responsibility but not as much as you're beating yourself up about. Doing so is simply uncalled for, at least at this point. Perhaps if you had known that you were going to be climbing a mountain, you would have brought more than a jacket and a water bottle.

Knowing exactly what you're up against is the first step to winning any battle, from WWII to your own personal battle of the bulge. There is more to reaching lifelong health than the right foods, exercises, and motivation.

So, what else is there? I'm so glad you asked!

I'm not talking about your emotions or how you link pumpkin pie to your late grandma. I'm also not talking about some breakthrough in the human metabolism. Believe it or not, it's much stronger than both of those issues. I'm talking about a force that drives millionaires, business owners, and blue-collar workers alike. It dictates almost every minute of our lives. I'm talking about **habits,** and they are far more powerful than we may have thought they were. They can literally make you or break you. They can pave your way, or make every effort for success next to impossible. Bad habits alone could be the very thing sabotaging your every diet attempt—and what an adversary they are. But hope is not lost. Before you tuck tail and hide, there is a way you can win this fight. There is a way you can flank your habits. You can arm yourself with knowledge of this dietary warfare, and have your bad habits on the run by the time the heavy artillery arrives. There is a proven method by which you can achieve healthy habitual patterns. You can control and harness the power of habits to achieve lifelong health. How? By re-setting your habitual eating and activity patterns so that, mentally as well as physiologically, you "need" to live a consistently healthy lifestyle.

What do you mean by "needing" to live a healthy lifestyle?

Have you ever known a person who seems to eat right and exercise year-round? Someone who consistently munches on health food and works out with so much vigor you would think they're actually enjoying it? In a world where yo-yo dieting and health fads are the norm, society looks at these types of people as if they're almost freaky. "Health Nut" or "Health Freak" are common terms describing those with this seemingly endless amount of motivation, discipline, and willpower. But as a self-admitted health freak, I'm going to let you in on a little secret. The idea that the world's fit share this unique and special discipline while the world's overweight share a major mental weakness is flat-out wrong. Those who consistently make healthier choices, day in and day out, do so for the very simple reason that they *want* to. They *crave* grilled chicken and vegetables in the same way you might crave nachos and beer. They find things like sugary, fattening foods just plain unappealing, or simply fear the consequences of how horrible these foods will make them feel. The healthy lifestyle has become such a deeply ingrained part of who they are that, for them, words like *relapse, cheating,* and *dieting* simply don't exist. Why? Because motivation has virtually nothing to do with it. They follow this lifestyle because it is their firmly established habitual pattern. Humans are creatures of habits. Habits give us comfort. It is only when we can control our habits that we can control our future.

Take heart—such habits can be learned!

Part One—

What Are Healthy Habits?

1—Getting Started

I've been on a constant diet for the last two decades.
I've lost a total of 789 pounds. By all accounts, I should
be hanging from a charm bracelet.   —ERMA BOMBECK

Introduction

What does the word "diet" mean to you? Limitation? Frustration?
Failure? It's interesting to me that we have transformed the meaning of
this word into something that makes us cringe. The original definition
of "diet" is "what is usually eaten," which can really mean anything.
It has only been the recent fad-diet craze that's given the poor word
a bad rap. Fad diets focus on making drastic behavioral changes at
a pace most people can't maintain. Because of this, traits such as
discipline, willpower, and mental toughness have been limelighted as
the secret to health.

Well, I'm here to tell you that, while important, these traits have
been blown way out of proportion. If you have failed before, it is not
necessarily because you lack these things. It is likely because you have
relied on them too much. Discipline and willpower are only temporary

fixes for the traits you'll need for a lifetime. The real secret is to develop the habits that will help you reach your goals. Habits shape our lives and rule our decisions, from how we dress to what's for lunch.

The reason why some people have sugar-loaded donuts and cappuccinos for breakfast is simply because they have done so for a long time. They're used to it, and their bodies expect it every morning and so they do it—every morning—it's a habit. Buying a new health book, no matter how good it might be, and getting all pumped up to make a different decision to eat something healthier the very next day is fighting a powerful, almost unbeatable, force—the force of habit.

In all fairness, it's not that these quick-results diet programs don't work; many of them do. You could lose weight and even gain muscle if it were possible to follow these programs to the letter. But it's not, and that's one of the reasons we are all still overweight. This overnight weight-loss approach puts motivation and willpower as the primary ingredients for success, placing you in a habit-versus-willpower fight and setting you up to fail.

We are what we habitually do, and any half-hearted attempt leads only to failure. We must be smarter than this. Instead of fighting against the power of habits, you must learn how to harness their power and make them work *for* you, not *against* you. The secret lies in taking the appropriate steps to gradually reshape your habits so that your body has a dependency on healthy living, similar to the way many people have a dependency on unhealthy living. A healthy body will be a mere by-product of gaining control over your habits.

Sounds good, right?

So, here you go again. Once more you find yourself taking a leap of faith and trying to jump back into the frustrating and often confusing world of diet and exercise. I don't know what made you decide to pick this book up and take it home with you. Maybe it was the colorful and creative cover, or perhaps the catchy title, or the interesting little blurb on the back of the book. What I do know is that you're probably not getting your hopes up just yet. Like the rest of us, you're probably tired of the whole "Get fit" situation. Yet you continue, month after month, year after year. You get back up, dust yourself off, and do it all over again. Why? Because even though your better judgment tells you there's no such thing, deep down you're hoping for a miracle, something that you can finally say *works!* Now don't worry, I'm not going to turn into some pessimistic trainer and tell you, "Sorry, there is no miracle." I'm not going to say miracles don't happen because I believe that, for many, the Healthy Habit Plan *is* that miracle they've been looking for all this time—and the craziest thing about it is that it's always been there, inside each and every one of you. It needs only to be unlocked.

You don't have to be super motivated or disciplined for my program to work for you. You don't have to already be fit or possess some type of mind-boggling mental toughness. Those are traits necessary for an elite athlete or an Olympian, not someone who just wants to be healthy. Nor do you need an incredibly high IQ, or an advanced degree in nutrition or exercise science to enjoy the benefits of the information in this book. All I ask is that you close your eyes, just for a moment, and try your best to wipe your mind free of all those past negative diet or exercise experiences; and while you do this, I ask that you extend your hand, so to speak, and allow me to take you all the way back to the beginning when words such as vegetables and exercise didn't bring about feelings of failure. If you look back far enough in your life, there was probably a time when running around or exercising seemed fun to you. Maybe there's even a memory when biting into a fresh orange gave you as much pleasure as that ice cream sundae gives you now. I know it's there somewhere because we were all born with an instinct to do and eat healthy things. Sometimes we just lose touch, and my job is to help you gain back what you once had.

"Why should I trust you completely?" you may be asking. I don't blame you for your hesitation. After all, asking everyone to close their eyes and allow themselves to be led down a different road often has people wondering, "Who's doing the guiding? And are they qualified?" Saying I'm qualified to change your life might seem like a bit of a stretch to you. In my career, I have found that the fitness industry has kept my ego in check many times. My first coach once told me, "Clients can always smell a rat." And perhaps that's where I excel. I ask you to trust me not by blind faith but by the sincerity of my voice, which I've always believed will come through. This is not the end-all, be-all of health and fitness, and I may not be the best trainer in the world, but this is my story of how I discovered a way to reach *hundreds* of people and to help them change their lives forever.

My name is Wes Cole, and I invite you on an exciting journey into a world where the battle of the bulge is won or lost in your head; a world where health nuts are not made, but reborn; a world where things like willpower and motivation take a backseat to what really matters: cultivating deeply ingrained habitual patterns that not only dictate your life but become a part of who you are. In this world you can learn to actually change the habits that derail your efforts, slowly guiding them toward health instead of misery. Move with me into an environment where people work out and eat right not because they should but because they *want* to, need to—a place where habitual health is real!

The Healthy Habit Plan Difference

My program can be considered a diet and fitness prequel, something that should be read before starting any health program. The cycles you will be learning about later in the book were designed as an excellent, standardized diet regimen, but the method can be applied to any approach you prefer. The Healthy Habit Plan isn't about bashing other diet or fitness philosophies. Whether you're a vegetarian or a self-described carnivore, you will find it fits into the grand scheme of the plan. If you prefer walking over weight training, it doesn't matter because ultimately, it won't affect your results. Love organic food? Great! Can't afford it? Well, that's okay, too, because you'll be just fine eating conventionally grown food. Think your body responded better to low carbohydrates than to low fat? Then that's fine. I won't debate with you on those choices because you know your body better than anyone.

Whether you're a Jazzerciser or a Jujitsu type of person, a boxer or a belly dancer, it doesn't matter because these are all just details, and oftentimes it's over-analyzing the details that will immobilize you. They call it "paralysis of analysis" when you have so much information thrown at you that you don't know what to do, so you freeze. "Eat low carb, but no, wait, low carb is bad so I should eat low fat . . . but wait, it's all about going vegan . . . oh, but maybe it's not about what I eat but *when* I eat." Then we get into the debate surrounding exercise, which is equally confusing. "It's all about cardio . . . but no, it's about weight training because that increases your metabolism, right? What about running because that burns the most calories . . . no, boot camp is the way to go now, right?" Thinking like this distracts you from what really matters.

So, what really matters? I'm glad you asked. You see, we live in an exceptional time. We now know more about the human body than ever before, and even though we all can get a little distracted by the mountains of inconclusive studies and claims, if we look hard enough, we find there is a lot of *conclusive* information out there, too. Details that are no longer theories but are very real facts. What the Healthy Habit Plan does more than anything is re-educate you from the ground up about *how* to pursue health—about your ideas of what health is and about having realistic expectations of yourself. I use scientific facts to address the real issues affecting your health. No pseudoscience, no theories, no maybes. My book lays down the facts about exercise and nutrition, brings you back to reality, and unclutters the mind from all the conflicting reports. This makes your fitness journey much more effective and enjoyable. I'm not saying that every health program you've been on before now was a joke. Most of them were probably good, but the Healthy Habit Plan contains the missing chapters that will allow you to follow the healthy lifestyle you prefer.

How to Use This Book

It is crucial that you don't skip any of the early chapters just so you can get to the cycles. Many of the techniques and philosophies used in the Healthy Habit Plan are based on scientific evidence. There is a method to all the madness, and I don't want you confused about the techniques in the middle because you skipped the beginning. You will just have to trust me here. After reading them in order, you will begin to understand why the book is laid out in this way. Each chapter and each cycle was designed to build on the knowledge of the previous one so that when you move through the cycles, you will be much more prepared and the journey will be as easy as possible.

Habit is either the best of servants or the worst of masters.

—Nathaniel Emmons

Your Five Biggest Questions Answered

Got questions? I have answers. The following questions are the most typical ones I receive from people who are hesitant to take that first step.

1. **What if I fail again? I'm afraid to even start.**

    I understand this question. You may have failed many times

before on other diets or health programs, but the Healthy Habit Plan has a very different approach. When I designed the Healthy Habit Plan, I had in mind the many people out there with very ingrained, unhealthy habits. Most other programs were designed for that small percentage of people who are able to develop new habits very quickly. Don't be upset if you're not one of them. A whopping 95% of people fail on their diets and health programs. You're not alone.

Unlike all the other approaches, we are going to move very slowly. The Healthy Habit Plan does not expect you to be a superman or superwoman. It was designed for people like you who have lost faith in the health industry and are unsure which way to turn. I don't expect you to have a tremendous amount of confidence at first. Confidence is something that will be developed along the way to achieving *habitual health*.

2. How is the Healthy Habit Plan approach different from other programs and books? What will keep me from quitting halfway through like I've done with all the rest?

Other health programs might be different from one another in content, but most are still very similar in their approach. They expect you to totally change your lifestyle, usually in about one day's time: weight lifting four days a week, on the treadmill another two days, and strange, new health food to top it off. You'll run across health experts who have the ability to inspire you easily and very effectively get you into action. Unfortunately, this is where they leave you. They don't teach you how to sustain your newfound motivation. So you strive toward your health goal with wild abandon before you realize just how powerful your established habits are.

This is not how the Healthy Habit Plan works. We attack one bad habit at a time so as not to overwhelm you with counting calories, carbohydrates, and fat grams all at once. The reason that health food might taste bad or boring to you right now is because you haven't yet developed the habit to enjoy these foods. By making small changes over many weeks, you will slowly introduce your body to healthy food and, eventually, you will crave brown rice and fish in the way you now crave hamburgers.

3. **How can I succeed if I get no support from my family, spouse, and friends to live a healthy lifestyle?**

Unfortunately, this is a common concern. People can be so uncomfortable with change that they don't even like to see it in others. Encourage them to join you, but if they don't, take the steps to find support elsewhere. In Appendix I of this book I recommend diet and support groups you can join. There are hundreds of such groups on the Internet, and there are dozens of online forums for personalized and specific support.

I list many tips in Appendix II to help you and your family prepare for your program, including asking family members to keep their unhealthy snacks in their private spaces, not in the kitchen.

Additionally, I am a big believer in group training and have found that small, independently owned aerobic studios and fitness gyms are the best at accepting and encouraging newcomers. Still feeling discouraged and uncertain? Sometimes you just have to put your foot down and stand up for what you feel is important. Focus on the people around you who aren't steering you away from your goal.

4. **What if I just don't care about my health that much? I
    don't care if I die early.**

    I firmly believe that no progress can be made unless you truly
    want it for yourself. Here is some food for thought, however:
    while you may not care about your life, someone else prob-
    ably does. Imagine the feelings of loss your wife, husband,
    children, parents, or friends will experience if you die early.
    You should also consider that people who abuse their bod-
    ies almost never die gracefully. Kidney failure, heart disease,
    cancer, and diabetes are all very painful diseases that can
    be directly related to living an unhealthy lifestyle. As you've
    likely heard or read before, there are things before death that
    are far worse than death itself!

5. **How can I get the quickest results? Your program seems
    very slow.**

    One thing I have learned is that very few people are able to
    stay on a typical health program long enough to replace old
    habits with new. You must understand that consistency is
    a critical ingredient. In fact, it is often more important than
    the program itself. I have been intensely researching healthy
    habits for years, and one thing I know, without a doubt, is
    that habits—even bad ones—are never developed in just a
    few days. Therefore, it will take you longer than a few days
    to alter them.

    Turn weakness into strength; the real secret to the Healthy
    Habit Plan is its slow approach. Since its introduction, peo-
    ple have called me saying that they have developed healthy
    habits within two weeks; others have called complaining
    about how long it took them to truly alter one particularly
    bad habit.

We're all different, but there is no way around the fact that altering habits is typically a much slower process than just a weight-loss or a muscle-building system. If you add up all the time you have spent trying and failing the many quick-results programs, you may realize that if you had been on the Healthy Habit Plan that whole time, you would have reached your goal and established positive habits to boot.

2—Going the Distance

Motivation is what gets you started. Habit is what keeps
you going.   —JIM RYUN

Babying Your Motivation

Things like motivation are often given the limelight as the secret
weapon in the fight to lose weight. Many of the fitness programs these
days read more like Tony Robbins than Dr. Atkins. Drill sergeant–like
trainers who yell, cuss, and scare you to run harder on the treadmill
often reach celebrity status. Motivational speakers sell out stadiums
and make millions on self-improvement CDs. Everybody wants to be
inspired. Everybody wants to listen to someone or to read books that
pump their soul with energy and positive thoughts. They want to ride
on the coattails of another driven individual in hopes of taking control
of their own lives and reaching their own goals. Seems like a good
idea right? Well, don't be so sure.

Before you dust off that *Rocky* soundtrack and head to the gym
in a blaze of glory, pushing yourself through a mind-boggling workout
relying completely on the whole "mind over matter thing," consider

this: deeply established habitual patterns have the ability to blast through your new, fresh motivation like a nail gun through soggy bread.

Because willpower and motivation are so overrated, this chapter will be one of the few places in this book where they will be mentioned at length. The perpetual myth is that the habitually healthy of the world have some type of unflinching willpower, stunning drive, and ironclad mental toughness that others don't. This is simply not true. Most health nuts have a secret: they *enjoy* working out. I mean, they don't even *feel right* if they don't hit the gym. It's a part of their life, just like brushing your teeth is a part of yours. They don't think about it, they just do it.

Healthy eating is the same way. There are people who actually prefer those vegetables and chicken breasts over a greasy, calorie-loaded cheeseburger. In fact, many couldn't eat the cheeseburger even if they wanted to because they wouldn't feel good afterward. Seriously! Try going a month without sugar and then go have a big ice cream sundae. It wouldn't work out well for you.

I'm not saying motivation is worthless. After all, without at least a little bit you wouldn't be reading this book. What I am saying is that we cannot fight our bad habits on motivation alone. It's guerilla warfare—we have to get dirty—and I'm going to make sure you have a lot of weapons, and that you know how to take care of them so you will always be ready for any battle.

After years of trial and error I have developed a method that one client described like this: "It's like you're cradling . . . almost babying my motivation." Exactly. The plan is to rely on techniques that spare your motivation, which will allow you to maintain consistency, and it is with consistency that habits are developed. Without consistency you wouldn't be able to subject your mind and body to a stimulus long enough for an adaptation, or habit, to be made, so being able stay on track is crucial—beyond crucial; it is everything. For example, the following are a few of the techniques we'll be using.

Small Changes

I've dedicated an entire section to this. It's not something you need to *do* but rather a mindset you must develop. The Healthy Habit Plan is not a get-fit-quick program; it's a habit-altering program, and this takes time. By slowly singling out one bad habit at a time, you will be able to put all your motivation and willpower on one thing. Like the karate master who uses his entire body to apply immense force on a vulnerable area of a much stronger adversary to defeat him, this is what we do with bad habits. The cycles are designed to have you inch your way to habitual health.

Unique Workout Principles

It has been my experience that solo workouts (working out alone either at the gym or at home) can often be the most mentally draining thing and can zap a newcomer's motivation in a mere couple of weeks. This is especially true for beginners because they have yet to develop the necessary skills to properly push themselves, and they don't understand proper exercise technique, which is a good way to get injured.

Home-fitness routines dominate the industry because there is a lot to sell. Treadmills, exercise DVDs, bikes, weights, and the like are big business. Unfortunately, most of these things end up being fancy coat hangers or just collecting dust on the shelf. Instead, my program teaches you to rely on motivation-sparing exercise methods, such as increasing labor-intensive activities or things that have to be done anyway (which are often referred to as "Have to's"). In addition, you will begin to understand the incredible benefits of group training and how to take back your health with traditional sports and active hobbies.

Enforcing a Positive Mental Connection

Before you understand the importance of developing a positive mental connection you must understand how damaging a *negative* mental connection is. If feelings of frustration, failure, deprivation, exhaustion, and boredom are the first things that come to mind when you think about exercise and dieting, then it should be no surprise to you that you haven't reached your goals. There's a difference between not really being in the mood to exercise and getting nauseous when you pull into the gym parking lot. There's a difference between being a little weirded out because you've changed your diet slightly and being in tears and ready to murder any fitness guru who tries to sell you another book because you've changed your eating habits so drastically!

The Healthy Habit Plan repairs your relationship with healthy living by making gradual changes, promoting sports and activities you enjoy, and introducing realistic gym-style workouts that give you a physical workout, not a workout of frustration. As you may know from previous experiences, losing weight and exercising can give you a great feeling of accomplishment. There's no better sensation than that endorphin-filled stretch-out after a long run or the filling up on a healthy dinner when you know you had other options.

What I am trying to do is develop in you *positive* feelings and associations with the things that will lead to better health. If positive feelings were the only thing that accompanied everyone's "Get fit" experience, then we would all be fit. Unfortunately, before we get there, we must overcome negative feelings we have unconsciously developed over the years. Things such as crash diets, impossibly hardcore fitness programs, and willpower-draining home workouts all contribute to these negative experiences, but we can do things to change this.

My goal is to make healthy eating and exercise enjoyable! If you're having fun, you'll want to do it more. And, naturally, when you do something over and over it becomes a habit. A healthy, positive relationship to your health program is the very essential soil in which habitual health grows.

The Power of Small Changes

Ninety-five percent of people fail on the typical fitness and diet program. This should come as no surprise, considering the way many of these programs are set up. Everyone is in such a big hurry! It takes years to become very overweight, *and years to take that weight off safely*.

My program, the Healthy Habit Plan, is quite simply a marketer's worst nightmare. What if I had put on the front cover **Get The Body You Want In Two Years!** or **Build Your Dream Body With Wes Cole's 8 Month Program!**? I didn't put that on the cover because you wouldn't have even bothered to look at it twice. *"Eight months? Build my dream body in two years? Is this guy on crack?"* That would be most people's reaction, but this idea isn't really that crazy at all. The idea that it takes a fair amount of time to get the weight off safely is completely logical considering that no one grew to an unhealthy size in just six weeks. It also makes sense that building muscle and developing the dynamite physique you saw on someone on the TV might not take months to achieve but rather *years*. I mean, do you really think that buff guy and shapely girl on that infomercial use the Ab-Blaster 2000 only twice a week, ten minutes a day? No way! These people have worked for years refining and developing their exercise and dietary habits to such a level that they can now maintain their lifestyle consistently. Perhaps they weren't even born with an incredible body and had to start slowly.

Let's face it—these days we live in an instant gratification society.

Most of us don't just want it now, we wanted it yesterday, and although modern technology has allowed this fantasy to become reality for a lot of things, true health is not one of them. The media and many fitness books utilize and sell quick-results programs because it's simply music to your ears. You have a beer belly or a baby belly and the reunion is in three weeks, so it's time to find a crash diet and show your old high school boyfriend/girlfriend that it was a mistake to break up with you in home room during your junior year! But just because this marketing technique gets you to buy these programs, it doesn't mean you will see the results you're hoping for.

The "overnight health nut" is one of the most pervasive myths in the industry. Your mind simply cannot go from 0 to 60, so to speak, without some serious psychological backlash. What this means is that you can't go from eating whatever you want to living on fruit, veggies, protein shakes, and discipline. You can't dust yourself off after being inactive since the Reagan Administration and start up a hardcore weight-training program four times a week. Just because you want to build new, healthier habits doesn't mean your old habits (the ones that led you into this mess in the first place) are going to instantly die. They're going to put up quite a fight because, right now, they're stronger. You've been making it a KFC night every Wednesday since you were in high school, so you can't replace that with a five-mile run and a vegan dish without some emotional consequences. That vegan dish was unfamiliar and unsatisfying, which means you end the day a bit tired from your run and a bit frustrated by your dinner. This does not create a positive connection to this lifestyle, thereby making consistency all that much more difficult. You see, your bad habits are stronger because you've been exercising them for a long time.

Interestingly, it probably wasn't always that way, no matter how much you hate physical activity now. You were probably active in high school or at least played when you were a kid. You may have slowed down in college, but I would guess you tried to stay fit to attract the opposite sex. But after that bi-weekly veg-out-on-the-sofa turned into three and then four times a week, you might not be doing anything more active than taking a shower. And your aversion to "healthy food" such as fruits and vegetables is nothing more than years and years of reconditioning your taste buds to enjoy stronger, more powerful flavors—the kind you would find in the Super Size Number 3 with a Coke. If you've spent the last eight years eating super-fattening, over-salted, or sugar-loaded foods after work each day, then it should be no surprise to you that steamed broccoli isn't going to tickle your fancy—but you can change that. You can get to the point where a candy bar tastes like putting two spoonfuls of sugar in your mouth and swishing it around: overly sweet, too rich, and simply not enjoyable.

A similar thing can be said for activity. I've had clients come in who hate exercise more than anything in the world, but then, in several months, they reach the point where they cannot imagine going a single day without exercise. Why? Because then they wouldn't feel good, they would feel sluggish, tired, or just not "right." For them, exercise has become a necessity, not something they thought they *should* do. You can be this way, too, but it takes time! The Healthy Habit Plan cycles are not short-lived. It may take months to conquer one bad habit, but when you do, it's over, it's taken care of, and you will never have to face that enemy again.

The Achievement Discrimination

Dietitians and trainers often face an uphill battle when striving to help their clients achieve real results by helping them change their habits. I find it interesting that most great achievements are won on hard work and time. Would a self-made millionaire's story sound as inspirational if you found out that he had just won the lottery? Of course not. We admire great achievers because it took not only hard work but *years* of hard work. Would a college degree mean as much to an employer if you had received it after only six weeks? What about a karate black belt in just two months? Probably not as impressive. Well, achieving an exceptional level of fitness or developing a strong body is just as challenging as many other great life achievements, especially if you have a long way to go. I'm not trying to discourage you; rather, I'm trying to sell my point, which is that your path to achieve your fitness is a marathon that you can win if you pace yourself. Don't bust out of the starting line in an attempt to sprint this road because it is too long for such a pace and you will fail. Change your mindset, and your road to health will be more effective and you'll enjoy the experience so much more.

Small Changes Work!

Don't underestimate the power of little health changes and what they can do for you. I'm not talking about the benefits being purely psychological, I mean real *physical* changes. Consider this: it takes a reduction of just 500 calories a day to lose a pound a week. This is two cans of Coke and a bag of chips. Reduce your cola habit alone, walk thirty minutes a day, or just get up and move around a little and you'll see changes. The best thing about it, if you continue with the new behaviors over a long enough time frame, you'll find yourself craving water like you once did cola and looking forward to being active. Sitting on the couch all day won't feel right, and a can of cola will end up tasting like pancake syrup. You will actually begin to *crave* a healthy lifestyle.

Greater Things to Come

More than anything, small changes allow for consistency and when you can actually have enough willpower to maintain something longer than two weeks, your new routine starts becoming more than just a new routine, it begins to mold into something different: a habit. You no longer need to tell yourself *"I have to be active today because Wes told me to."* You do it without thinking because it's a part of your day now. Motivation is not a factor anymore. This is what I like to call "non-motivational consistency," and it is the beginning of altering your habitual patterns.

In my years as a trainer, the number of fitness newbies who could jump into a killer fitness routine and a dramatically different nutrition program virtually overnight are so few that I need only one hand to count them—and I have fingers left over! This is the reality of accomplishing your goals: anything worthwhile takes time and it also takes work. If it didn't it wouldn't be special. Six-pack abs wouldn't be a big deal if everyone had them. If achieving a healthy body weight was easy, we wouldn't be discussing it right now. It's hard work, but by taking the right steps, slowing down and following my approach, you can make it much more pleasant and actually obtainable.

What Is Change?

One of the reasons I believe so many nutrition programs fail these days is a simple philosophy that many people share: moderation. It's the idea that you can do everything you've been doing, just scale it back a bit. It seems on paper to sound reasonable because, after all, life is all about balance, right? You can eat anything you want; you can have that candy bar or cheesecake or soda, just less of it. Does this sound appealing to you? Of course it does! Things like "Eat the foods you love and still lose weight" or "Everything in moderation" have been on the list of favorite subtitles for diet programs over the past twenty years. Why? Because it's marketing genius. People want to believe they can achieve their goals without changing their lifestyle. The idea that one can still party, still drink, still eat chocolate cake, and still have gallons of soft drinks all while achieving fitness goals is on top of everyone's wish list. What moderation really says to many is "live the lifestyle you want, but just tone it down a little."

So, you've turned down the volume, but what you really needed to do was change the station. Instead of two candy bars, you just have one; or instead of a whole large pizza, you just have a whole medium pizza. Well, you may have toned down your bad habits a bit but you haven't replaced them with anything good or beneficial, so you're left feeling dissatisfied or, even worse, deprived. Soon enough, you're back to two candy bars and a large pepperoni.

Just so we're clear on this point: scaling back your bad habits is not the same as *changing* them. That's one of the secrets behind the Healthy Habit Plan. Every time you are required to eliminate something bad or unhealthy, you are allowed to replace it with something healthy. In this way, you never feel deprived. Sure, there's a bit of an adjustment but that's what change is about; you are making a difference in your health and your life.

Some Healthy Truths

So, you want the truth? Can you handle the truth? Maybe not, but just like a Band Aid stuck to skin, sometimes you just have to rip it off quickly so it will hurt less. Stay with me while I get some unpopular truths out on the table for you to consider.

1. **You can have a wild night life OR a healthy body.**

    In my entire career I have never worked with anyone who can drink and party every weekend and still achieve his or her health goals. Furthermore, if you're the type who feels that it would be impossible to go an entire week without drinking, then you *do* have a dependency on alcohol. Dependency on alcohol is not okay. Also, realize that if you drink a lot, worrying about carbs and protein and cardio is pretty pointless. Bottom line is you need to pick one: a healthy body or a wild nightlife.

2. Be prepared to permanently give up at least one bad food.

This is crucial to the habit-altering process. To develop mental sensitivities to new foods or their replacements, you have to stick to it for at least four to six weeks. You can't eat healthier food twice a week, off and on, while still eating your normal foods and expect to refine your habits. Developing physical sensitivities to things such as sugar or fat requires avoiding that food entirely for a certain amount of time. This is possible to do because we pick only one bad habit at a time and we conquer it for good. By the time you're done with Cycle One, you will have not only lost your craving for sugar but also your tolerance of it. It will taste overly sweet; the texture won't be as inviting, and eating too much of it could cause severe discomfort. This is what makes the Healthy Habit Plan truly foolproof. You will stay on your health program because you physically have to and mentally prefer to, but constantly allowing "cheat days" or even small portions of forbidden foods in the cycle retards the habit-altering process and prevents good habits from forming.

3. Being active every day is not obsessive.

When I'm asked how often we need to be active to make it a habit, people often look at me like I'm obsessive when I say "Every day." But I'm not obsessive at all. You can vary your intensity, of course, but the human body was designed to be active *every day,* not just Mondays and Fridays or Tuesdays and Thursdays. Thirty minutes of moderate activity daily is enough to see some changes, but most important, it's the quickest way to make it a habit. If you think you're too busy to do at least something active on a daily basis, then you need to adjust your priorities. The average American watches more than four hours of TV a day, so saying you don't have time is very unlikely. You must retrain your thinking if the idea of being active every day is extremely foreign to you. The Healthy Habit Plan has a very flexible and very realistic approach to exercise. There are many guidelines designed to prevent burn out, maintain motivation, and provide for an overall positive exercise experience.

4.   You must be honest with yourself.

Most people know immediately whether or not a diet or exercise program they're about to start will be realistic for their level. The Healthy Habit Plan not only strives to give you the truth but also forces you to be truthful with yourself. What is the truth? The truth is you're probably not disciplined enough to work out on your own, and your willpower, when it comes to bad food choices, is probably not strong enough to avoid them. You're probably not yet ready for super-intense workouts despite your athletic achievements in high school, and you do probably eat more than you think you eat.

It is not my intention to be mean, and I definitely want to give people the credit they deserve, but in this Tony Robbins or Zig Ziglar–like mindset in which we live, merely believing in oneself has been likened to invincible armor. Unfortunately, this is not the case. Believing in yourself *is* important, but you also have to be realistic. Belief without consistent action is about as effective as just hanging that motivational poster on your wall, and that lack of consistency can lead to a serious case of denial.

In my experience, gyms are full of overweight people who truly believe they can maintain consistency all by themselves, even as they're signing the cancellation slip. There are plenty of people who have failed diet after diet but truly believe they're disciplined enough to get on the next extreme nutrition program. Unfortunately, belief doesn't always transmit into success. They find themselves confused because they clearly show discipline at work but somehow have trouble saying no to the office birthday cake. This path we're beginning together is about priorities and it's about being truthful. Having belief in yourself is important but it's only a piece of the puzzle. Having a good game plan, re-working your priorities, and admitting your weaknesses are the first steps.

It is my opinion that moderation simply doesn't work for those who are just beginning a diet regimen. Allowing small amounts of forbidden foods throughout the week will only retard the habit-forming process and lead to few positive outcomes. Most moderation-based health programs turn quickly into half-hearted programs with little or no lasting results. That one cookie you were allowed turns into one and a half, then two. I know, you tell yourself "I'll have two today and I won't eat any tomorrow," but then tomorrow comes and your stomach is growling and that cookie (or cookies) look so good.

The fear many people have is this: They can't imagine going the rest of their lives without cake, some beer, or some bad food. To them, life wouldn't be worth living this way. If you see it like this, then I encourage you to look at it in two alternative ways. 1) The Healthy Habit Plan is not about never having that piece of cake again, it's about changing your habits so you don't even *want* that piece of cake. 2) Moderation can work but only for the people who have *already* established healthy patterns. They can do this because their habits will protect them. Even on holidays when you are surrounded by tons of temptation, you will instinctively go for the healthy options, not because you need to but because you will prefer it. You may think I'm calling for a life of total abstinence, but you'll find that when you alter your habitual patterns, things change, simple as that. There might be things in your life that you'll say good-bye to forever but by then, you won't mind at all.

A habit cannot be tossed out the window; it must be coaxed down the stairs one step at a time.

—MARK TWAIN

I hope that you are starting to understand what my points about living healthy are all about. It's about developing habitual patterns that will let you enjoy healthy eating and exercising. It's about developing simple awareness and educating yourself as to what and how much you're eating. It's about realizing that turning around a bag of food and actually reading the calories contained inside the package before you eat it isn't that inconvenient.

It's about breaking free of denial and realizing that you don't have the discipline to work out alone at home. It's about standing on that weight scale a couple times a week and accepting the fact that you're either improving or not and, more than anything else, it's realizing that deep down inside, *you already know* why you're in bad shape. You know it's not your thyroid, you know it's not because you don't eat often enough or that you're hitting starvation mode. You know it's simpler than that. Your habits of inactivity and eating too much have been practiced so much that now they are instinct. It feels normal for you to eat when you're not hungry, it feels great for you to eat unhealthy food and to not work out for a month, and basically, your habitual patterns go against the laws of proper body weight and health.

You know it's just this simple: you have to find a way to eat less and move more. Unfortunately, we all know this is easier said than done. Habitual patterns are like an old, faded-but-embedded tattoo. It can be removed but it's not going to be easy. I believe that the cycles of the Healthy Habit Plan effectively address and overcome this problem, and will lead you through constructive change.

3—Facts or Myths?

The chains of habits are generally too small to be felt until they are too strong to be broken.   —Samuel Johnson

The Real Deal about Meal Frequency

The idea that one must eat every two or three hours in order to lose weight is the biggest hoax the diet industry has spewed out since the chocolate diet. I have enough data dating back to the 1980s that clearly proves meal frequency has no effect on your metabolism. A University of Ottawa study, led by Eric Doucet, showed that frequent small meals didn't promote weight loss. Participants consumed a reduced-calorie diet with meals served either three or six times per day for eight weeks (total daily calorie intake was the same). Both groups lost about 5% of their body weight, but the frequency of meals had no effect on weight loss or metabolism. When the calories are the same, the weight loss is the same regardless of meal timing (Cameron et al. 2010). With that said, I'm going to challenge this old style of health and weight loss by addressing some of its major problems.

It's outdated—

Science has been slowly catching up with the multi-meal approach and recent studies make you wonder how this technique became popular to begin with. A study published in the *British Journal of Nutrition* stated that meal frequency has no significant impact on the rate of weight loss during caloric restriction (Verboeket-van de Venne and Westertep 1993). The theory behind frequent feeding is that the more you eat, the more you digest and, thereby, the more calories you burn digesting. Not to point out the obvious, but your body is digesting because you consumed *more calories*.

Your metabolism is directly related to the number of calories you consume, otherwise known as the thermic effect of food or TEF. What this means is that when you eat a small meal, you have a small metabolic response, and when you eat a larger meal, you have a larger metabolic response. If you're eating five or six meals a day, each meal has to be small (otherwise you're not dieting) so the effect of these meals is on the smaller side. And, again, if you have only one or two big meals a day, you will have a much larger TEF response per meal because you've ingested more calories in one sitting. If you're thinking, "Okay, which is better?" then you're missing the point. Science shows us it doesn't matter. The amount of calories you eat does affect your metabolism, but how you break them up is irrelevant. It's the *total daily calories* that matter.

Eating all the time is inconvenient—

Our North American society is built around breakfast, lunch, and dinner. However, if you were in a different country, perhaps a European country, you would probably find the two meals a day approach more comfortable. The important thing to keep in mind here is that in the beginning of any lifestyle change, you need to find ways to make starting and maintaining the lifestyle as easy as possible. Remember, a beginner's motivational fuel, no matter how potent it might seem, has its limits. A beginner should be focusing on the *big* reasons they are overweight. High-sugar diets, unhealthy carbohydrate addictions, inactivity, lack of health and fitness education, and simple denial about how much they really eat are the main factors.

Whether you are eating once, twice, three, or ten times a day doesn't matter because science shows us that how often you eat does not aid in weight loss. It's the total calories that count, but let's just say that the grazing method seems like it might work for you. It doesn't matter, right? As long as calories are the same. You're right, but it has been my experience that packing, managing, and eating the correct portion of foods every two or three hours can be very impractical, time-consuming, and difficult to maintain long term. For anyone other than some elite body builders and friends of mine who are career athletes, I have never personally found this approach to work well in the long run. Life just gets in the way. A late day at the office, a sick baby, a family reunion over the weekend, and suddenly the time you used to pre-pack and stock up on all your mini-meals is gone. And we all know that the vending machine is not really a smart alternative.

> ### Habit Helper—
>
> *Now, there is some validity to the idea that certain foods will boost metabolism more than others simply because the amount of energy it takes to metabolize the food is relatively high in relation to the number of calories it contains; however, that boost is small and very temporary. At the end of the day, it's not a method on which to solely rely.*

Some evidence suggests that the human digestive system was never designed to be constantly digesting and eliminating food, and that long periods without food are best so that it can rest. This is supported by tremendous studies documenting incredible health benefits from intermittent fasting or restricted calorie diets. The studies have received well-deserved attention in the last couple of years because of results such as increased insulin sensitivity, stress resistance, reduced morbidity, and increased life span (Anson et al. 2003).

Bottom line, changing your health status isn't easy because it means you have to change your lifestyle, and although many don't want to hear that, in reality it was that very lifestyle that led to being overweight in the first place. Because of this we must go about changing things slowly, and most important, making things as simple and convenient as possible in the early stages. So, for most people, life and work are set up for three meals a day: breakfast, lunch, and dinner, making it the simplest and best approach.

Habit Helper—

Remember: protein doesn't build muscle, food builds muscle. Protein is just part of the equation. Weight lifters can save money when it comes to expensive protein shakes because their bodies can absorb only so much at one time and the extra calories (even protein calories) will still be stored as fat.

It's based on the marketing and supplement industry—

Any approach to dieting should be looked over with a fine-tooth comb, particularly when the diet is part of the weight-loss industry where there is so much money to be made. The sports supplement industry loves the frequent feeding approach because no one has time to cook five or six times a day. So what do you do? Hmmm . . . how about some protein shakes or meal replacement powders? I find it to be an odd "coincidence" that the regimen of multiple meals a day became popular around the exact same time that all the new protein companies emerged. Don't get me wrong: there is nothing bad about having a high-quality protein powder in the cabinet; I mention this just as food for thought when you run across a trainer, diet guru, or supplement salesman who is pushing the frequent-feeding method. Very often, the people who support this idea have protein shakes, meal replacements, or their own line of nutrition bars ready to sell you. I don't, and never will, have my own line of supplements. I have nothing to gain, no money to make, by recommending a normal meal schedule. It's just what makes the most sense to me.

Some good news about frequent feeding—

I had the privilege to interview one of the winners of the show *The Biggest Loser* a couple of years back. Danny Cahill told me that the frequent meal schedule helped him control his hunger and eventually allowed him to lose a record amount of weight. On the other hand, my brother, who had dealt with an eating disorder in the past and was extremely thin, found that it was impossible to take in all the calories he needed in just three squares a day.

Even though it is rare, I have recommended a more frequent feeding method to some clients when there is a particular reason to do so. People who are hypoglycemic or who have diabetes or other disorders might need to eat more frequently to maintain blood sugar levels because their bodies respond differently from how others' might respond. Certain college athletes and professional fighters with whom I've worked in the past have told me that eating frequently keeps up their energy.

So before you read this chapter and say, "But, Wes, this worked for me!", understand that the purpose of this chapter isn't to prevent you from eating frequent meals; rather, it is to teach you that meal scheduling is a matter of personal preference and of achieving your personal goals. An active college football player looking to put on muscle is going to have goals that are different from the goals of a thirty-seven-year-old mother who wants to lose twenty pounds and who works forty hours a week. Weekly scheduling will also differ. A construction worker might find eating two times a day more convenient than the computer technician who prefers frequent fueling because he works at his home several paces from the kitchen. Different strokes for different folks. If this works for you then I say, "Go right ahead" but, if you're trying to lose weight, don't forget the added responsibility of making sure those small meals stay small.

Science is clear when it comes to meal scheduling. ***It doesn't matter!*** Whether it's five times a day, once, or twenty, at the end of the day you either ate too many calories or you didn't. As you go about changing your health, you must understand what worked for your friend might not work for you. You are unique physically and mentally. Find a meal schedule that fits your lifestyle and that requires the least amount of willpower from you.

The Myth of Meal Timing

You've probably heard this caution: Don't eat late at night or it will be stored as fat. The logic seems sound. At night, you're less active so eating a large dinner will put weight on you, but this is simply not true. There has been no scientific data proving there is any relevance to meal timing as far as weight loss is concerned (MacMillan 2008). The human digestive system is truly incredible, absorbing a lot of nutrients and regulating itself throughout the day. "The time of day a person eats is not as important for overall weight gain as the amount of calories eaten during the day," agrees Jeannie Gazzaniga-Moloo Ph.D., R.D., a spokesperson for the American Dietetic Association. If you require 2,000 calories per day to function normally and you give your body those 2,000 calories, then that's the important part. The timing of those meals (or meal) is irrelevant. Your body is smart enough to figure out how to regulate that energy intake with its energy expenditure. Now, if you're eating 2,400 calories (400 more than you need), that's when you run into trouble.

For the sake of argument, I am going to mention a study conducted by Northwestern University in Evanston, Illinois, showing a correlation between meal timing and weight gain. Before you get too excited about it, however, I want you to actually look up the study and read it top to bottom. The study was conducted on two groups of mice and looked at the effects of eating during different phases of the circadian rhythm, or internal clock. Our internal clock is what tells us it's daytime or nighttime and adjusts our metabolism accordingly. One group of mice was fed during the daytime and one group during the night. Now, mice are nocturnal so it is normal for mice to eat during the nighttime hours but not during the day, the opposite of humans. At the end of the study, the day-fed mice did gain more weight than the night-fed mice but not for the reasons the headline would have you believe. According to the study, the day-fed mice were consistently less active than the night-fed group over time, indicating a decrease in energy expenditure. Furthermore, the day-fed mice consumed slightly more than the night-fed group (Arble et al. 2009). So, the mice that gained weight did so because they ate more and moved less.

I can't express to you how important it is to do your own research and read these studies through. Very often the headlines are misleading for marketing or attention-grabbing purposes. Always, always, always *read* them! Educate yourself! Don't be a victim of some creative author's headline-writing abilities.

Redefining Hunger

By now I hope you can see past the myths associated with dieting and exercise. Things like "muscle loss" or "increased metabolism" shouldn't scare or excite you like maybe they used to. And I hope that any type of abdominal machine or exercise gadget that you see on a 2 a.m. infomercial doesn't have you running for your credit card. You know the overnight health nut approach is simply a myth, and that it takes time to not only build a healthy body but to also establish the right habits that will allow you to keep it. You're not afraid to get on the scale and check your progress, and you know that physically losing weight and getting healthy really boils down to this simple fact: move more and eat less.

What I'm going to talk about in this section is something that on the surface might seem like a real physiological issue: hunger. The word "hunger" is scary for many people—so much so that an entire industry of shakes, between-meal bars, drugs, frequent-feeding diets, and supplements have been created to prevent that horrific feeling of hunger. Before I go into how to deal with it, I need to define what hunger really is. The reality is that for most people like you and me, hunger is, and always has been, a psychological issue rather than a true biological event. Associating your hunger with true starvation is ridiculous especially when you sport a good ten to fifteen pounds of extra padding around the middle. It is true that a host of complex, hormonal responses happen when one eats that make us feel good, and there's nothing wrong with enjoying this feeling. One of my favorite pleasures in life is eating dinner with my wife. It soothes me emotionally and physically, but when one starts to become obsessed with the pleasure that food brings, then there's a problem.

How does one battle this addiction with food? This is, of course, a complex issue, but I assure you there are ways around it. Although I am not overweight, I do love eating, and I love food as much as any obese person does and so do many healthy people despite the myth that thin people are "anti-eating" or "anti-food." The difference is that I have learned to find pleasure in other things as well, and it's critical to understand that what you feel at noon—that uncomfortable feeling like you have to have food—is nothing more than a mental response. You eat at this time every day and so your mind expects it. It might send you fake, subtle signs telling you that you must have food now, but I promise you they will go away after a few minutes. Why? Because it is not a *physical* need. It has been well documented that the human body can live for months without food. Do you really think your body *needs* lunch because it's been two hours since your sausage cheese biscuit? Come on! I'm not telling you not to have lunch, but when these "illusions of hunger" start to pop up as you begin to reduce your calories, remember they are not real. It might take some focus, but you'll get accustomed to it. Here are some ways to help you learn how to deal with counterfeit hunger.

- *Wait ten minutes before getting seconds.*

- *Drink a full glass of water before and after your meal.*

- *Have a breath mint or mint gum. (Mint has been proven to reduce appetite.)*

- *If it's suitable to your palate, try eating something spicy before several of your weekly meals. Certain studies indicate that spicy foods are a natural appetite suppressant.*

A Note on "Starvation Mode"

Since we've been talking about hunger, I'd like to address another myth that seems to have transformed into fact in the public mind: it's called "starvation mode." It's the idea that if you go too low on your calories, your metabolism will shut down, forcing your body to digest muscle and to store fat. The human body can survive for months without food—only a few days without water but *months* without food. Do you really think your metabolism is going to shut down or that your body is going to start digesting healthy muscle tissue over fat just because you skipped breakfast and have been without food for three hours? That's not going to happen, unless you have been chronically underfed for a long period of time. It has been well documented that there is no drop in human resting metabolism until seventy-two hours without any food (Chan et al. 2003).

What's interesting is that "starvation mode" has become the ultimate weight-loss excuse. Years ago I conducted a little experiment at my gym with new clients. They were all overweight, roughly fifty pounds or more, and I found that more than 90% of them shared the same belief that their metabolism is just slow, causing their body to hold onto fat. So, long story short, they believed they were overweight because they *weren't eating enough,* and that their body's metabolism was sabotaging them by going into "starvation mode." This kind of thinking just shows you the power of marketing. The media has actually convinced overweight people that they're overweight because they are *under* eating, when in fact eating *too many calories* is the real problem.

Bottom line, starvation mode (at least in this aspect) is a myth. Simple as that. It doesn't exist. There is no proof. The time has come to give it up. If you're on a diet and feeling hungry, then understand it just means that you want to eat. You are far from experiencing starvation, and to think that you're starving because you've cut 500 calories from your daily intake or because you went to bed without dinner is an exaggeration. True starvation is when you've tapped out *all* your fat reserves and your body is digesting muscle and organs. It is one of the most painful ways to die that exists today. Still don't believe me? Well, consider this: Have you ever seen a fat starving person on one of those infomercials or in a world news report? I haven't.

I want you to understand the point I'm trying to make. Let's be clear as to what starvation is, and stop using the phrase so loosely. Given the reasons you are reading this book, it's probably safe to say you are fortunate and not experiencing starvation.

A Realistic Approach to Organics

Since we've been discussing healthy eating, you may be thinking, "Why not use all *organic* food on the Healthy Habit Plan? That would be so much better and make me have results even faster, right?" Well, maybe not. I am going to answer some common questions that may make you feel just as good about eating conventionally grown foods as you used to feel when you walked into your local organic market.

1. **If I buy organic, won't I be supporting all the small-scale organic farmers in America?**

    Not necessarily. Unless you're buying directly from your local farmers' market (not the organic supermarket), the majority of what you purchase actually comes from a large, likely well-known, corporation with a big profit margin. Trader Joe's, a popular organic food store, made close to 4.5 billion dollars last year. Unfortunately, except for the occasional, small-town farmers' market, gone are the days of the organic food industry being controlled by the old, friendly farmers—at least mostly. General Mills owns the organic food brand Cascadian Farm, and Kraft owns Back to Nature and Boca Burger. Your favorite cereal company, Kellogg's, owns Morningstar Farms, and out of the 1 billion dollars in produce sold at Whole Foods in a recent year a mere 16% was locally grown (Howard 2009).

    Bottom line, if you're eating organic food just to help out the local farmers, you need to make sure that what you're buying actually came from them. After doing so, in most areas of the country you will find that the selection is rather limited, leaving you no choice but to buy from a larger corporation as well. If you look on the bright side, however, large corporations often employ a larger number of people, so by supporting them you are doing your part to help these people support their families, too.

2. Isn't organic food safer and more nutritious than conventionally grown food?

It would be awesome if super healthy and safe eating were as simple as buying organic. However, the USDA and the FDA have stated, "there is no evidence to support the idea that organically grown foods are safer or more nutritious." Even more frustrating is the fact that, without the presence of mild preservatives, organic foods have been shown to spoil faster (Rhosey LLC 2006).

The most important thing to remember when it comes to food safety is the handling of your food. Always wash all fruits and vegetables regardless of how they were grown, and cook all meats to a safe temperature. While all methods of farming have been guilty of contamination, an independent study by the University of Minnesota showed that organically grown produce was contaminated with the *E. coli* bacteria five times more often than conventionally grown produce (Morano 2004). This is chiefly due to the widespread use of composted animal manure as a fertilizer.

The most nutritious foods are those you grow yourself or those you buy directly from a local farmer. Local is the key. All produce, regardless of farming methods, begins to lose nutritional value from the moment it is harvested, so the faster it makes it to your table, the more nutritious it will be.

3. Isn't organic produce pesticide free?

Unfortunately, this is simply not true. Contrary to what you see in the media, organic food is not entirely pesticide free. Many natural pesticides are used, all of which pose the same theoretical—but remote—dangers as synthetic pesticides. For example, two very common organic pesticides are Pyrethrum and Rotenone. Pyrethrum is rated by the EPA as a "likely human carcinogenic" and Rotenone has been shown to cause symptoms of Parkinson's Disease (Avery 2001).

The point to remember here is that these natural pesticides, as well as synthetic ones, break down very quickly, so residue, if any remains at all, is microscopic and well within levels safe for human consumption. So even though fruit may absorb the pesticides during the growing process, the amount present would be similar to only one drop of food coloring in the Great Lakes.

4. Wouldn't it be better for the future of people and the planet if everybody ate organically grown foods? I've heard that organic farming is the "green" way to go.

I agree that we could all be a little greener but organic farming right now is incapable of yielding enough food supply to feed the world's population. Even if every farm on the planet converted to organic farming, there is the potential to feed only two-thirds of a population that is still increasing. High-yield conventional farming has demonstrated time and again that it has the capability to feed a massive and growing population. I think we can agree that feeding people is the first step in ensuring their future. Some may argue that the planet itself can handle only so many people, however, so making a massive population boom possible is not the best idea for the future of the planet. There is a balance that needs to be found between feeding the world and saving it.

Whether or not a larger population would be detrimental to the planet is beyond the scope of this book; but from a humanistic approach, all human beings deserve to be able to feed themselves and their families, which means we need to support forms of agriculture that allow that to happen.

Have you ever heard of a man named Norman Borlaug? He easily could be labeled as one of the greatest human beings who ever lived. Borlaug was a genetic scientist who discovered how to triple wheat and rice production at a critical time when food supplies in Mexico, Asia, and Latin America were desperately low. He was the father of the "Green Revolution" and is said to have saved more than a **billion** people from starvation (Easterbrook 1997). Borlaug had this to say about organic farming, "I've got quite a few shades of green in me. Not the extreme green that some of these who operate on cloud nine have. When people are suffering from hunger, you have to make certain choices . . . There are 6.6 billion people on the planet today. With organic farming we could only feed four billion of them. Which two billion would volunteer to die?" (Borlaug 2000, 2010).

Dr. Borlaug's legacy has been carried on through teams of scientists who understand that the world in which we live is changing rapidly. Everything from medical treatment to computers have benefited from scientific advancements. Yet when it comes to finding ways to produce more food for the growing number of hungry mouths, many folks seem to be unwilling to apply the same beneficial technology. In this country, we are lucky not only to have an abundance of food but also an abundance of choices. While I would never discourage anyone from buying and eating only organic, I would certainly never judge anyone who supports conventional, high-yield farming either.

So, pound for pound, the nutritional value may be the same. Success with this program is possible regardless of the source of your healthy food choices. In this day and age, where you obtain your foods has become a philosophical, economic, political, and highly personal decision.

Chapter 3 References

Anson, R. Michael, Zhihong Gua, et al. 2003. "Intermittent Fasting Dissociates Beneficial Effects of Dietary Restriction on Glucose Metabolism and Neuronal Resistance to Injury From Calorie Intake." Proceedings of the National Academy of Sciences of the United States of America. April 30. doi: 10.1073/pnas.1035720100.

Arble, Deanna, Joseph Bass, Aaron Laposky, et al. 2009. "Circadian Timing of Food Intake Contributed to Weight Gain." Northwestern University, Evanston, Illinois. *Obesity* 7, no. 11 (May 5). Published online September 3, 2009.

Avery, Alex. 2001. "The Deadly Chemicals in Organic Food." Center for Global Food Issues. www.cgfi.org. Originally published in the *New York Post,* June 2001.

Borlaug, Norman E. 2000. "Ending World Hunger: The Promise of Biotechnology and the Threat of Anti-Science Zealotry." *Plant Physiology* 124 (October): 487–490.

Borlaug, Norman E. 2010. "The Green Revolution Revisited and the Road Ahead." Special 30th Anniversary Lecture. The Norwegian Nobel Institute. Oslo, Norway, September 8.

Cameron J.D., M.J. Cyr, and E. Doucet. 2010. "Increased Meal

Frequency Does Not Promote Greater Weight Loss in Subjects Who Were Prescribed an 8-Week Equi-Energetic Energy-Restricted Diet." *British Journal of Nutrition* 103, no. 8 (April): 1098–1101. Epub November 30, 2009. PubMed PMID: 19943985.

Chan, Jean L., Kathleen Heist, et al. 2003. "The Role of Falling Leptin Levels in the Neuroendocrine and Metabolic Adaptation to Short Term Starvation in Healthy Men." *Journal of Clinical Investigation* 111, no. 9 (May 1): 1409-1421.

Easterbrook, Gregg. 1997. "Forgotten Benefactor of Humanity." *Atlantic Monthly* 279, no. 1 (January): 75–82.

Howard, Phillip H. 2009. "Organic Processing Industry Structure." Michigan State University. June. www.msu.edu (accessed May 24, 2010).

MacMillan, Amanda. 2008. "Relax—Your Holiday Health Concerns Might Just Be Myths. Myth: Eating at Night Makes You Fat." CNNHealth.com (December 18). www.cnn.com (accessed June 10, 2010).

Morano, Marc. 2004. "Does Organic Food Have Higher Levels of Fecal Contamination?" *CNS News* (June). www.organicconsumers.org (accessed June 3, 2010).

"Norman Borlaug: Father of the Green Revolution—He Helped Feed the World." 2010. ScienceHeroes.com. www.scienceheroes.com (accessed June 3, 2010).

Rhosey LLC. 2006. "What Does the 'Organic' Label Really Mean?" USDA-FDA Nutrition Labeling. usda-fda.com (accessed October 3, 2011).

Verboeket-van de Venne, W.P., and Kester Westertep. 1993. "Effect of the Pattern of Food Intake on Human Energy Metabolism." *British Journal of Nutrition* 7, no. 1 (July): 103–115.

4—Tips to Keep You on Track

A habit is something you can do without thinking—
which is why most of us have so many of them.

—FRANK HOWARD CLARK

The NEAT Principle

NEAT is an acronym used by exercise geeks that stands for Non Exercise Activity Thermogenesis. To sum it up, it's basically a person's activity pattern outside the gym or beyond the scope of classical exercise. For example, a heavy-labor construction worker's NEAT level will almost always be higher than that of a computer technician. Avid gardeners who spend a lot of their free hours planting, digging, and tilling will have higher NEAT levels than people who go home and play video games.

Here's how it works. A study was conducted by James Levine of the Mayo Clinic with two groups of people: obese sedentary people and lean sedentary people. Neither group participated in an exercise program. What the study found was that *lean* sedentary people were standing or were ambulatory for 152 minutes longer per day than obese sedentary people and, similarly, the obese group sat immobile for 164 minutes longer than the lean group. The study then postulates that if the obese subjects adopted the same posture allocation as the lean subjects, they could expend 350 additional calories per day because of the energy cost of standing/ambulating (Levine 2006). Additionally, this caloric expenditure almost identically matched the caloric expenditure identified in an earlier study by Dale A. Schoeller of the American Society for Clinical Nutrition. Schoeller looked at the the formal exercise level that obese people need to adopt in order to promote negative energy balance and weight loss (Schoeller 2003).

So what does the NEAT principle have to do with you? Science has come to the conclusion that how active you are outside the gym is just as important as how active you are in the gym. There is even a theory that one of the reasons weight training and traditional cardio programs work is because they give people more energy, so when they leave the gym they do more things. They go shopping, walk the dog, or mow the lawn. They feel stronger and healthier, and the end result is more calories burned through activity, not just exercise.

Let me give you a true-life example of the NEAT principle in action. Several years back I found and adopted a stray Labrador mix that had been hit by a car. She seemed like a pretty laid-back dog . . . until she got some much-needed weight back on her and her leg healed. She became a four-legged terror, destroying everything in sight. I talked to the vet, and he said the solution was simple: walk her for half an hour every day.

Now, I work in a gym six days a week, and if I'm not teaching martial arts, training clients, or working out myself, you'll usually find me with my feet kicked up watching reruns of *Seinfeld*. The last thing I wanted to do was walk a dog, but sometimes you got to do what you got to do.

It was hard coming home late from work or getting up early to walk that mutt, but after a while it became a habit and I actually reached the point where I enjoyed it. But here's something I didn't expect: over the course of about a month, I started to notice my weight drop a bit. I didn't fret and just suspected it was due to water loss, but altogether I had lost about eight pounds. I hadn't increased my exercise in the gym, and, in fact, I was taking it easy because of an elbow injury, so I didn't understand where the weight was going. I thought about my calories and was scratching my head until I realized the answer was licking me right on the hand the whole time. It was the walking! Now, I know what you're thinking—you're a fitness expert and you didn't realize that? No, I didn't because it didn't *feel* like exercise. That's the beauty of it.

My Lab and I have since parted ways—we gave her to a relative who lived in the country—but I'll never forget the lesson of NEAT that dog showed me. It's the simple principle of calories in, calories out that had been drilled into my head by teachers and professors for years, but after decades of high-intensity cardio and heavy weight training, my mind had become clouded and missed the simple principles that NEAT had to offer. Let's review these points so that no matter what fitness level you are at, you'll never forget this important principle and what it does.

It teaches us that high intensity exercise is not necessary—

At least for initial weight loss or for reaching a basic level of fitness, this is true. If you stay extremely active while gardening, doing sports, playing with kids, or cleaning, you can maintain or even lose body fat as long as your caloric intake stays the same. Simply finding ways to stand up while doing activities you typically sit down for can be a great start.

For all those who think you must puke in a bucket or wheeze like an asthmatic to get fit, you're wrong. A study conducted on an Amish community showed that even while eating a diet rich in fat and calories, both men and women in the community maintained a very healthy weight. Why? Because their daily activity level was so high. The men reported an average of ten hours of vigorous activity per week, and the pedometers they wore indicated that the men took more than 18,000 steps per day and the women took more than 14,000 (Bassett et al. 2004). The women cleaned all day and prepared food for the evening meals, while the men gardened and built and maintained the properties; but here's the thing: it wasn't always super-intense activity. Sure, they might have sweated a little but not always. It's just that their activity was constant—meaning from sun up to sun down—and most important, *consistent.* They got up and did it again . . . every day.

Many fitness experts want you to believe that you have to be willing to pass out to get in shape. Well, that depends. If your goal is to be the next ultimate fighting champion, then, yes. If you want to sign an NFL contract, then, yes. But if you just have a little weight to lose and want to get healthier and stronger, then the answer to fitness might be all around you in less-intense but more consistent activity.

NEAT activities take less motivational fuel—

What better way to develop a habit and to get in shape than doing things you have to do anyway? When was the last time you walked your dog, washed the car, cleaned the house or the attic, or built your kid that tree house you've been promising? It won't cost you a dime, and just think how clean and fixed up everything will be. These activities won't burn as many calories as a group training class but they all add up. Just like you can nickel and dime your way into the poorhouse, you can inch your way to a healthy weight. I have since incorporated what I like to call "Have to" chores or tasks that you have to do anyway. Not only does this burn calories, it also helps break little "bad" habits such as watching TV for four hours on Saturday while eating a whole bag of chips or zoning out on the computer.

Even though I found a new home for my dog, the two years that I had her instilled some major habits even in me. I said good-bye to those *Seinfeld* reruns a long time ago, and no matter how tired I feel after work, my wife and I almost always go on a little after-dinner walk.

You eat less—

Chances are if you're moving more, you're eating less, and this is a big benefit because there is a huge connection between mindless eating and watching TV. Think about it: when was the last time you watched TV, surfed the web, or played video games without munching on anything? If you didn't, you're one of the few. Making a conscious effort to increase your NEAT levels will automatically reduce your calories.

It clears up confusion—

A lot of people in the health and fitness industry want to confuse you about why you might be overweight or unhealthy. Maybe it's a malfunctioning metabolism, or you're probably vitamin deficient. You don't eat often enough; maybe you eat too much red meat or too much bread. It seems like every move you make or calorie you eat is wrong. So how on earth are you ever going to lose weight? You want the real truth? The million-dollar answer? Here it is: You have to find a way to move more and eat less. We are all different from one another, and we can all do different things to achieve that goal. You might like to eat six small meals a day, or just one. You might like group training or working with your trainer, or you might hate the whole gym scene and want to focus on a sport, hobby, or something to get you moving more. It doesn't matter what you do, but learning how to increase your activity *entirely,* not just in the gym, can help anyone from the housewife to the pro athlete, and NEAT shows you that it all matters, even the little things. *Your* little things might be gardening or walking, or they can be watching TV and eating bonbons. Either way, it will add up.

NEAT can really work but, in my opinion, it should be only one tool in your arsenal. Developing a habit for more intense exercise is the best bet, but any activity is a good addition. During this gradual addition of activities, watch out for the effect it may have on your appetite. A study published in the *American Journal of Clinical Nutrition* showed that people often increased their calories right after a workout, often by enough to negate the calorie burn of the workout (Pomerleau et al. 2004). Remember, when I was walking my dog I had not changed my dietary habits one way or the other. If I had, the results would have been different. With a good food diary and a no-guessing policy, you might be surprised at how healthy you can become by just doing the things you need to be doing anyway.

Home Workouts: An Oxymoron

Working out at home; such a thing sounds cool—so modern, and so convenient. Why get in your car and fight the traffic, search for a parking spot, and deal with the crowded gyms when you can simply work out in your underwear in the privacy of your own home with your brand new Solo-Blaster 4000, or your Ab-Blitzer? It sounds so appealing, which is why currently the home fitness market is absolutely booming. The U.S. fitness equipment manufacturing industry has more than 100 companies with a combined annual revenue of more than three billion dollars (Hoovers 2010). These are the sales even before the equipment reaches the middlemen who slap on a retail price (often double or more what they paid) and then sell it to you. Internet shopping is in full swing and with only a few clicks of your mouse—you don't even have to leave your house—you can have a brand new exercise machine delivered right to your door with a computerized personal trainer, twenty different interval workouts, special jelly-cushioned pads to make it easy on your knees, and all the other fancy trimmings that made you want to fork over a couple grand. And why not? With a good piece of cardio equipment, a rack of heavy dumbbells, and maybe a pull-up bar and a bench, what else do you need to get a full body workout? After all, a gym membership will end up costing you more in the long run, right? And working out at home sounds so great because you don't have to worry about the big meatheads secretly smirking because you're one of those "two-plate guys." You don't have to worry about some creepy guy hitting on you all the time, and best of all, you don't have to be social. You've worked all day, dealt with people all day, so the last thing you want to do is drive to a packed gym and walk around a big free-weight area pretending to be friendly and trying with all your heart to look like you know what you're doing.

I've literally grown up in the fitness industry, and I've seen thousands of people get on workout programs. I watched many succeed but I've watched many more fail. Over the years I've learned a lot, and I've been around the fitness block a time or two, so to speak, so I'm going to tell you something that might upset you or that might make you nod your head up and down and say, "He's right." **Home workouts don't work!** There, I said it. I don't care how

> **Habit Helper—**
>
> *Don't get roped into the idea that if you build a ton of muscle, you will burn a ton more calories. Muscle does burn more calories than does fat but not nearly as much as previously thought. According to Dr. Robert Wolfe at the University of Arkansas, don't believe pie-in-the-sky claims that a pound of muscle burns a whopping 50 to 100 calories a day. A man who does strength training three times a week for six months, for example, may gain four to six pounds of muscle. That would result in 20 to 48 extra calories burned a day— not much, considering that you need a deficit of about 500 calories a day to lose a pound a week (Berkeley Wellness 2010).*

convenient they sound, how much more comfortable you might feel working out alone, or how much more affordable they might end up being—they just don't work.

It's as if an engineer came up with a perfect schematic of a project on paper but it just didn't play out when people started actually trying to build it. It's still a failed plan, no matter how pretty the plastic scale model or prints looked.

There are millions of Americans who have fancy treadmills and steppers draped with clothes, Ab-gizmos stuffed in closets, and dumbbells thrown in the corner of the garage collecting a thick coating of dust; and there are millions more who will go right back to the computer and search for, and often purchase, the next big thing when it comes to fitness equipment. They collect and collect, yet the only weight they've lost is in their wallets.

Albert Einstein, among others, has been credited with saying that the definition of insanity is "doing the same thing over and over again and expecting different results." So why do you keep purchasing more and more home fitness items when you have thousands of dollars stuck in closets already? Because you keep searching in hopes that one of these machines is surely going to get you in shape, when the reality is that none of these pieces of equipment failed you but, rather, it is the *home fitness strategy* that failed you.

Despite massive failure rates, the home fitness industry keeps pumping out new pieces for you to buy, and you often do. Let's go over a couple of common myths as to why many people fall into this fitness strategy.

Myth 1—It's more convenient.

Not really. When I first started training, I set people up for home workouts. Traveling all across town, I would check up on them every month or so. At that time in my life, I had fairly high drop-out rates, and these clients never saw results. I went into a state of denial for a while, pretending to be confused about why it wasn't working, but a little guy inside my head was screaming at me every time I would set someone up on a program. That voice was screaming *"There's no way this is going to work!"* I don't know how many times I would be trying to train a client and the phone would ring and ring and ring, sometimes ten times. UPS would always seem to know when I was there because they would always have a big package to deliver right during cardio.

Animals are great; I love them and they love their owners, but they don't like you ignoring them so you can move a large object up and down. I spent most of my time trying to keep big Labs from jumping on my clients when they were trying to do push-ups or squats. I would let them outside or put them in another room at my clients' request, and nine out of ten times they would wreak havoc and break something. The little dogs would frequently get spiteful and do their business right on the rug in front of their owners to show their disproval. Yes, this trainer has picked up plenty of dog crap.

Then the phone rings some more while the neighbor is knocking on your door because the Lab you just put out has hopped the fence and is chasing his cat. Then the baby wakes up. He simultaneously screams, spits up, and fills his diaper within seconds of opening his eyes. Barely five minutes into cardio, my client has been interrupted three or four times, and we're just getting started. Then the husband comes home. He's had a bad day, and the last thing he wants to come home to is some weird guy in the living room. "Who are you?" he says. "I'm the trainer," I say awkwardly, while waiting for my client to quickly change the baby's diaper. Then the husband sees the wife and gets angry because she forgot that they have the Joneses coming over for dinner in one hour. Long story short, the session is canceled for another more convenient day.

This is a true story of one of my earlier clients. I did go back to that woman's house for training sessions; but it wasn't much different.

She was interrupted many times, and if I wasn't pushing her every step of the way, she wouldn't have had a chance. This woman didn't succeed; she didn't lose a pound because she never really got to work out.

This is just one example of what happens to many people even though they truly believe that working out at home is more convenient. I don't train people at home anymore no matter how much money they want to throw at me. I don't do it because I know they won't succeed, and if they don't succeed they don't hire me ever again.

Myth 2—Working out at home is more practical.

I know what you're thinking: "If home workouts aren't that practical then why are there so many companies, books, exercise DVDs, and products that cater to the home workout?" Well, it's all about the mighty dollar. For many people their home is their castle, their fortress of solitude from the outside world. People you're uncomfortable with or don't like, never get a chance to come into your home. After a hard day's work, where do you go to relax and depressurize from the noisy, cruel world? Your home, and this natural nesting instinct that we almost all have, is what makes the idea of working out "in the privacy of your own home" so appealing.

The marketing behind the billion-dollar home fitness industry depends on this desire to be home. They know that doing a workout at home sounds not only more convenient to you but also more comfortable. This is especially true for fitness newbies who feel self-conscious about being unfit as well as insecure about their lack of knowledge on how to exercise. Most of the fitness products advertised on TV, whether it's some kind of new tread climber or abdominal gizmo, were never intended to be marketed to the already fit. The reason for this is that the majority of fit people get their exercise outside the home and, in that case, how did they get fit in the first place? The same way they stay fit, by stepping outside their little sanctuary. It doesn't matter what they do, they might sign up at some gym and lift weights, run with friends, take up cage fighting or Jazzercise, or engage in any number of other calorie-burning activities.

You see, the home is not the proper environment to get an adequate workout, and it's not just because of all the possible distractions. It's because your mind associates the home with a place to relax, eat, unwind, and watch TV—not as a place to exercise. One of my clients owned a computer business for which she had to hire employees who could do their jobs at home. She said that only about one person out of a hundred had the type of personality that allowed them to properly work in the home environment and be able to stay with the company. Work has a totally different type of motivation. It's stronger than most motivations because it's in the same category as paying bills and keeping up with your mortgage. So here's my point: if it takes a special person to stay motivated working at home to get a paycheck, how can average people maintain enough motivation to properly push themselves to exercise with any kind of intensity or consistency in this non-conducive environment? The answer is that they can't, and the massive amounts of home fitness stations that are less than six months old and being resold on eBay, thrown in closets, or used solely as a four-thousand-dollar coat hanger prove it.

"You're wrong, Wes, I work out at home!" Okay, well, I didn't say it was impossible. Some rare people can do it, but before you write me off as a complete nut, let me ask a couple of questions.

What does "I work out at home" mean? Are you still working out at home? Do you work out consistently because if you don't, it doesn't count in the pursuit of building healthy habits. Dusting off the old bench press in the garage when the weather is nice and your college buddies are in town doesn't count as a home workout program. That's just goofing off. If your definition of working out at home is to pull out your groovy, solo-fat machine from the closet because your girlfriend's pissing you off and you need to "let off some steam," that's not a home fitness workout. That's just a temper tantrum. There's nothing wrong with goofing off or letting off steam in a responsible, respectful manner—keep your home fitness equipment for those occasions—but I want you to recognize that these uses don't in themselves make up a consistent workout habit.

If this does not describe you then I commend you for being a rarity, and I wish continued success to all the serious "cellar dwellers" on their exercise programs. If this does describe you, however, then it's time for a new strategy. It starts with reading, understanding, and eventually believing that the following statements are true:

- *I've tried working out at home and it never works for me, so I'm changing my strategy.*

- *I've already spent too much money on home exercise equipment I'm not using, so I'm going to stop!*

- *I will not be afraid of stepping outside my sanctuary.*

- *I'm not going to consider myself an introvert or anti-social (because all fitness newbies are introverts and anti-social in a gym).*

- *I know the Healthy Habit Plan was specifically designed to make sure I have a **positive** workout experience, so I trust it.*

Read this again and again and understand that I won't let you down!

How Not to Be Afraid of the Scale

Don't weigh yourself. Throw the scale out. See how your clothes fit instead. Muscle weighs more than fat anyway so weighing yourself doesn't matter if you lift weights. What does all this mean? Over the years I've heard a lot of excuses for why many people refuse to weigh themselves and, despite what they may say, I know the real answer. Most of them simply don't like what they see. A lot of people who are heavy don't frequently—or ever—weigh themselves, which contributes to allowing a few pounds to accumulate here and there over the years. Then, once they do weigh themselves, they are often surprised by how much weight they've gained. They get on a typical diet and do it half-heartedly like most people do, guessing their calorie intake, exaggerating the caloric burn of exercise, and basically just kidding themselves.

> **Habit Helper—**
>
> *A 2006 study from Cornell University found that college freshmen instructed to weigh themselves every morning gained almost no weight during the school year compared with a 7-pound gain for those who weren't given a scale.*

Never underestimate denial; it is why many 300-plus-pound people truly believe with all their hearts that they don't eat much at all. You can lie to yourself, you can lie to your trainer and your dietitian, you can pretend to diet, you can get bigger clothes so they look baggy and feel more comfortable, and you can get the latest diet book of the month. You can breeze through five minutes in that $3,000 elliptical machine and feel good, like you did something for your health. But the scale is the barest of all truths. It reminds me of a famous line a boxer once shared: "cheat on your road work during the dark mornings and you'll be discovered under the bright lights." The scale doesn't lie.

You can tell yourself that your twice-a-week hit-and-miss attendance in an intense water aerobics class put ten pounds of muscle on you, or that the scale is cheap and inaccurate, or that you're retaining water, but deep down all that's going through your mind as you step on the bearer of truth is that moment of lapse when you gorged on a half gallon of Häagen-Dazs or took down six pieces of pizza because it was late and your coworker brought it to the office.

Many people hate the weight scale because it's a fitness version of a report card. My father, who was also my martial arts instructor, once told me, "You're never standing still in your martial arts training, you're either going forward or backward; you're either giving it your all or you're not." I look at achieving fitness in the same way, and you must recondition how you feel about weighing yourself.

What do you call the type of people who obsessively, every morning after going to the bathroom, weigh themselves? Is there a name for those fanatical people who take notice of a five-pound weight gain after that long liquor-filled Cancun vacation and immediately begin to cut back on calories? Those people who seem to closely watch the scale and keep tabs on it? Yes, there is a name for these supposedly anal-retentive souls: they're called thin people. According to Dr. James Hill and Dr. Rena Wing of the National Weight Control Registry, a study among individuals who have been able to successfully maintain long-term weight loss showed that 75% of the participants weighed themselves frequently. Dr. Hill states, "Frequent weighing may therefore serve as an 'early warning system' for these people. I suspect that when they have gained a few pounds, they implement strategies to prevent further weight gain. . . . Other studies have found that self-monitoring predicts success in long-term maintenance of weight loss" (Hill and Wing 2003).

It's a fact that people who weigh themselves daily are more likely to successfully be able to maintain a healthy body weight. Why then do diet gurus all over the country continue to tell us to do the opposite? First of all, the reason Captain Diet Guru of the month is telling you this is because it's something he knows you want to hear. It is a popularity contest that you fall for. I don't care about being popular. Instead, I have an undying desire to get you lean and healthy, and I'm telling you that *you need to weigh yourself every single day!*

Why does becoming obsessive help? Simply because it's a constant reminder. When you see someone who is very heavy, with fifty-plus pounds to lose, this is something that didn't take a year or even two years to gain. This took more like eight or ten years to gain; slowly but surely over time adding a pound here and there until one day Mr. John Doe wakes up and says, "What the heck? Where did this belly come from?!" If he had been weighing himself daily he probably would have noticed at some point, "Hey, wow! I'm putting on a little weight!" Back then if he had addressed the problem, he would have had ten or fifteen pounds to lose, not seventy. Maybe not easy but certainly not impossible. He could have cut back a little on his intake, become more active, and he would have been back to a healthier weight in a relatively short time.

Why should you weigh yourself? Because it's a lot easier to lose fifteen pounds than it is to lose fifty. With the scale, weight gain can't creep up on you, it's right there staring you in the face. Be brave. I understand it will be discouraging at first, but you will get used to the scale being an encouraging motivator rather than an unpleasant nag. Think of it as "Okay, thanks for the reminder!"

The Power of Discomfort

Every holiday season, millions of people in this country put their new diets "on hold" until after New Year's. Yet why do the Habitually Healthy remain strong throughout? How can someone do this? To begin thinking about this, consider that the fear of mental, and especially physical, discomfort can often be more powerful than your biggest craving. For example, many people say there is no amount of willpower in the world that will keep them from eventually giving in and gorging on their beloved sweets! Are they right that it is unavoidable for everyone? Not when you change your habitual patterns! I assure you there are no sugar addicts out there who will feel the same about sweets after having gone through six weeks on a sugar-free cycle only to suddenly re-introduce chocolate donuts back into their diets. I even prove this to you by letting you try those once-beloved unhealthy foods at the end of each habit-altering cycle to show you how your body has adapted to healthy living.

I have explained what it takes to have a healthy body, and that is living a healthy lifestyle. Short-term diets are based on willpower and motivation and often do nothing to alter your habitual patterns. This is because they take the "everything in moderation" approach, or they start you off at such an advanced level that you can't maintain true consistency. Allow me to say it again because it is such an important point: habits don't rely on motivation and willpower. They rely on other things, things that don't sound nearly as glamorous but are far more effective in the long run. Reduced cravings and physical rejection of unhealthy food are some of the factors forcing people to remain eating in a healthy manner. One of the biggest reasons is mental and physical discomfort. The reason I don't eat many unhealthy foods that are available is because I don't crave them anymore or they simply don't taste good to me anymore. But, what about the unhealthy foods that I do still like or crave? I still have to stop myself because I know that, if I eat more than a little bite, I won't feel good. I don't mean just a mental response like guilt; I mean physical responses such as stomach cramps, anxiety, lethargy, or nausea. I eat the way I eat because it makes me feel good and not because I am immune to all temptations, because I'm not.

When you develop true healthy habitual patterns, you will

instinctively be careful about what kind and how much unhealthy food you put in your mouth. The habitually healthy are some of the few who can use portion control in a very effective manner because they fear what will happen if they go overboard. People do what makes them feel good both mentally and physically. Now, whether this "feel good" habit is smoking or an aerobics class is up to you and your habits. Make no mistake, though, you will do what you habitually do, simple as that. The power of discomfort is one of the biggest reasons why habitual health followers continue their lifestyle.

If you have truly developed a habit for healthy foods, then most of your favorite "bad foods" won't even taste good to you anymore, and even if you do still enjoy their taste a little, you will eat only a small amount knowing that over-indulgence will lead to painfully discovering what the difference is between a proper portion and overkill. This is the only way portion control really works. I'm here to tell you that no matter how much of a junk food addict you might be now, if you slowly introduce your body to nutrient-rich healthy foods, your body will learn to like them and will become increasingly sensitive to sugars, fats, and preservatives and, eventually, you will not be able to tolerate them at all.

Now, we've talked a lot about diet but what about exercise? You will experience strong withdrawals if you develop a habit for activity and then suddenly stop. There are days when I simply don't have time to exercise and don't even want to, but I do it anyway because I will experience nervousness, lethargy, depression, irritability, and poor concentration if I don't. Just ask anyone who knows me. I work out even on Christmas morning because I have to! Understand that you can teach your body to need and even enjoy exercise every single day of the year. No willpower or discipline required. When you reach this point you will follow this lifestyle of healthy living because you will feel awful living any other way. This is the absolute raw power of habits.

Chapter 4 References

Bassett D.R., P.L. Schneider, and G.E. Huntington. 2004. "Physical Activity in an Old Order Amish Community." *Medicine and Science in Sports and Exercise* 36, no. 8 (August): 1447. Author reply 1448.

Berkeley Wellness Alerts. 2010. "Gain Strength, Lose Weight: Claims vs. Reality." February 16. www.berkeleywellnessalerts.com (accessed June 18, 2010).

Hill, James, and Rena Wing. 2003. "A Focus on Obesity, Part 2." *Permanente Journal* 7, no. 3 (Summer). The National Weight Control Registry. xnet.kp.org (accessed 2010).

Hoovers: A D&B Company. 2010. "Industry Overview: Fitness Equipment." First Research. www.hoovers.com (accessed May 31, 2010).

Levine, James A. 2006. "Non-Exercise Activity Thermogenesis." *Proceedings of the Nutrition Society* 62: 667–679. doi:10.1079/PNS2003281.

Pomerleau, Marjorie, Pascal Imbeault, Tonney Parker, and Eric Doucet. 2004. "Effects of Exercise Intensity on Food Intake and Appetite in Women." *American Journal of Clinical Nutrition* 80, no. 5 (November): 1230–1236.

Schoeller, Dale A. 2003. "But How Much Physical Activity?" *American Journal of Clinical Nutrition* 78, no. 4 (October): 669–670.

5—The Nuts & Bolts

Habit is a cable; we weave a thread of it each day, and at last we cannot break it. —HORACE MANN

The Stages of Habit Development

You've read the philosophy and understand the importance of gradually introducing your body and mind to the healthy lifestyle. You understand the limitations of motivation and the importance of maximizing or "babying" your motivational potential. You are beginning to understand how to avoid a negative mental connection to your new lifestyle. What comes next is an overview of the stages of habit development, each linked to a cycle in the program.

You'll experience all four motivational stages in each cycle. For example, you'll go through stages 1 through 4 in the course of Cycle One, then again in Cycle Two, and so forth. Here are the stages of habit development:

1. **Inspiration/Motivation**

    This is the spark that initially gets you to want to change

your life. The beginning of the Healthy Habit Plan instills inspiration and shows you how to develop and baby your motivation. This leads you to start looking into, or to show *interest* in, ways to achieve your goal.

2. **Interest—**The two levels of interest are:

Contemplation

This is where you start doing research into possible ways to achieve your goal. You're buying that book, listening to fitness advice, and really thinking about your own path to health.

Action

This is where you have made up your mind about which path to take and you are ready to take action! You have done your research and are ready to apply what you have learned.

The Healthy Habit Plan + Action = Confidence

3. **Confidence—**When real confidence in healthy living is established, it contributes to the development of two traits critical for habit development:

Positive Mental Connection

This happens when you have started to eat healthy foods and to be active, and you have seen results. You are starting to feel better and look better and you attribute that to the healthy lifestyle you have adopted. This is the very definition of developing a positive mental connection. For the first time, the thought of healthy food and exercise brings about *good* feelings and, when this happens, it is human nature to want to repeat it over and over again to keep having those good feelings. You have made yourself proud and have some awesome results to show for it. This leads to non-motivational consistency.

Non-Motivational Consistency

What this means is that you are consistent with eating right and exercise, not because you feel like you should but because you want to, because doing so brings about those good feelings. Once you are consistent for a long time, sure enough, you reach the final step and that is a *habit*.

4. Habit

Finally, healthy living has become second nature to you. While you're busy living your life, unbeknown to you on a conscious level, you are staying consistent and maintaining your health. Now, you only understand life with healthy food and healthy activity. No small feat, you should congratulate yourself!

Get Ready for Success

Wes Cole's Healthy Habits was designed for anyone who wants to live a healthy lifestyle consistently, but especially for the millions of failed dieters and fitness enthusiasts who, one way or the other, stopped short of achieving their health goals. If you are one of these people, the reason you may have fallen short has more to do with your approach to health than any character flaw. It's not realistic to get on a high-intensity fitness routine if you haven't been active since the Reagan Administration.

You must understand that if you are sincerely interested in changing your health, you don't need to train your mind to get on a diet and "trim down" or hit the gym and "tone up." Say those common phrases to yourself and really analyze what they suggest. Those phrases scream *"Temporary"* and that's exactly how most diets are set up. If you want to really improve your health you have to be ready to change your life. In order to do this, you will need to prepare yourself and your environment for success.

Nine Tips for Making It Work

1. **Do not make your exercise regimen too intense, too soon.**

   Do only the activities you enjoy. The same goes with your diet. Eat the kind of foods you enjoy while still complying with the rules of the cycles. There are healthy versions of any kind of food.

2. **Remove only the forbidden foods in your particular cycle from your house.**

   Don't start tossing out every single bad item in your pantry and replacing it with something healthy; this will freak you out and you will likely want to quit the program. Remember, gradual introductions.

3. **Read about health and fitness a lot; subscribe to some of the health magazines.**

   Become educated in the subject (if you're not already) and learn what exercise and eating right are doing for your body. Even if you are savvy about how food and exercise contribute to your well-being, continuing to read about it serves as a daily reminder and encourages you to consider new research and points of view.

4. **Reinforce your motivation point, no matter what it is.**

   If you're motivated by the social benefits of appearing trim, healthy, and attractive to others, take note of the inches or pounds you have lost and reward yourself with each victory by purchasing a new outfit or something that makes you feel good about your appearance. If you're motivated by a health scare or doctor's warning, continue to educate yourself on the risks of an unhealthy lifestyle and the benefits of eating right and exercising. Check back in with that doctor or other healthcare professionals to receive further feedback and support that you're on the right path.

5. **Planning is the most powerful way to develop a habit.**

   Plan your meals, snacks, and activities ahead of time. Last-minute planning is the most harmful setback to your motivation, especially in the beginning. It's also why so many people fail when trying to stick to their diets.

6. **Surround yourself with positive energy and people who believe in you and understand your goals.**

   Be prepared for even your closest friends to unintentionally sidetrack you. They don't always mean to, but competing with my clients' friends and families is one of my toughest jobs, and I don't always win. Keep in mind that people can be very uncomfortable with change and many times don't even like seeing it occur in others.

7. **Incorporate activity and exercise into your life.**

   Move away from thinking of physical fitness as a twice-a-week session. Our bodies were designed to be active every day. Do something physical every day, with varying intensities. This is the quickest way to develop a habit for exercise.

8. **Don't have total "free" days! I mean, don't allow yourself days off in which you can eat anything and/or do nothing.**

    You will end up feeling worse after consuming too much unhealthy food or not being active enough, and you can do damage to your good habits.

9. **Make eating and physical activity a social, fun thing.**

    Meet with friends for a walk or a competitive tennis match. Make eating special again. Take up cooking; sit down with friends and family and enjoy your food and each other. Stop focusing on large portions and quick, low-quality foods.

Get to Know the Four Habit-Altering Cycles

The Cycles at a Glance

I developed the step-by-step Healthy Habit Plan during the years of owning a gym and training clients in the joys of creating good habits. These four cycles are the steps you will take to defeat your old, unhealthy habits and replace them with new ones. They are dietary and activity guidelines that will gradually, but absolutely, change your life. The dietary guidelines include detailed descriptions of the specific foods I want you to either avoid or to add to your meals, and their effects on the body. The activity guidelines show you what activities are allowed and *not* allowed for each cycle.

The beauty of the habit-altering cycles is that you're eliminating only one bad habit at a time, starting with sugar. As the cycles progress, they build on one another until lean meats, vegetables, whole grains, and fruits become the fare you crave for dinner. To reinforce the lessons learned, each cycle ends with a habit test.

The habit tests are designed to gauge the strength of your new habits, and the results will determine when you are ready to move on to the next cycle.

The fitness guidelines correlate with the dietary guidelines, slowly increasing in the amount and frequency of activity until your body literally begins to crave exercise. Unlike programs that immediately immerse you in challenging physical exercise in either members-only or home gyms, my program begins with simply performing daily chores that are very physically active, and progresses through the cycles to the point at which hard workouts are the norm. These cycles also have a frequently asked questions section and a physical activity habit test.

Next is a quick reference guide to the habit-altering cycles.

Cycle One—6 weeks

Nutrition

Eliminate processed sugar, including "hidden" sugar in foods; fight sweet cravings by replacing processed sugar with naturally occurring sugar, such as in fruit (but not juice) and sugar-free sweeteners.

Fitness

Do what-you-already-do; physically challenging activities, such as lawn mowing, building, cleaning, dog walking, or any general labor activity. These are also called "have-to" chores.

20 to 30 minutes daily.

Cycle Two—6 weeks

Nutrition

Focus on carbohydrates and proteins in the right amounts.

3 weeks: carbohydrate and protein mixing

3 weeks: switching to healthier carbohydrates or starches

Fitness

Moderate-level group training classes in traditional gym settings *OR* participate in a favorite sport or moderate-level activity, such as dancing or basketball.

2 times a week minimum in addition to your "have-to" chores.

20 to 60 minutes at a time.

Cycle Three—6 weeks

Nutrition

Get rid of saturated fats and trans fats. Reduce the amount of sodium you consume. No eating at restaurants.

3 weeks: eliminate trans fat and reduce fats, for example, by trimming it from meat.

3 weeks: reduce sodium

Fitness

Upper-level group training. Consider competitive sports.

Participate in events such as city and charity runs. You can hire a personal trainer starting at Cycle Three.

3 to 4 times a week in addition to your "have-to" chores.

30 to 60 minutes at a time.

Cycle Four—6 weeks

Nutrition

Learn how to write down and calculate the calories in everything you eat. Educate yourself and be aware of what's in your food.

Fitness

Standard twice-a-week weight-training workout. Continue with competitive sports and physical hobbies such as karate, hiking, hunting, and so forth. You should feel the need for some type of daily exercise by now.

3 to 4 times a week for 30 to 60 minutes at a time.

Part Two—

The Four Cycles

A nail is driven out by another nail. Habit is overcome by habit. —DESIDERIUS ERASMUS

6—Cycle One

Creativity can solve almost any problem. The creative act,
the defeat of habit by originality, overcomes everything.

—GEORGE LOIS

Cycle One Nutrition: Sugar Reduction

Cycle One duration will be at least six weeks.

To Do—

- *Stop consuming all forms of added sugars.*

The goal in Cycle One is to increase your body's sensitivity to all kinds of concentrated sugars. All refined *and* natural concentrated sweeteners, such as sucrose (table sugar), corn syrups, fructose sweeteners, as well as molasses, maple syrup, and honey will be replaced with low-calorie or calorie-free sugar substitutes. I recommend the natural, low-calorie approach to sugar substitutes, such as Stevia, but that particular brand is not required.

I'm here not to dictate which type of sugar substitute you should use, only to tell you that Cycle One is all about substituting sugar. There are differences among the replacements, so experiment with the many brands on the market today. Talk to your friends or visit your favorite health food store and ask for a few recommendations. (Refer to the Review of Acceptable Sweeteners, pages 101–104, for a complete list.)

> **Habit Helper—**
>
> *The goal in Cycle One is to increase your body's sensitivity to all kinds of concentrated sugars (even if they're natural). Remember, it is not about killing your sweet tooth—only replacing bad sweets with good ones.*

This is not a total-carbohydrate reduction phase, so natural sugars in foods such as whole fruit and milk, as well as starches like potatoes and bread *are* allowed. Juices of any kind will not be allowed, though, because of their unnaturally high fructose content.

I do realize that many natural sweeteners, such as molasses and honey, contain some vitamins, minerals, and antioxidants, but they are also very high in sucrose content (some equal to or greater than regular table sugar) and are often just as harmful to your health overall as refined sugars. I've found that when I attempt to wean my clients off of some of the most common and harmful sweeteners, such as white table sugars or corn syrups, they attempt to satisfy their initial sugar withdrawal with unusually large amounts of natural sweeteners.

The goal in this cycle is for your body to develop a general sensitivity to all refined and natural sugars, and to teach your body to learn to enjoy them au naturel, that is, in the form of various fruits.

In short, stick to foods that either you already know have no sugar or to foods labeled with these words: sugar-free, no sugar added, or diet. Steer clear of foods whose labels tout "reduced sugar," as these still contain some amount of added sugar. Become a label reader! While you're reducing sugar intake, increase the amount of time you spend reading labels and examining them for hidden language that translates to "sugar."

You may encounter items, such as canned tomatoes or milk, that have a small number of grams of sugar *but they may not be from added sugars!* If you see an item that says it has "some" sugar, read the ingredients. Although the item contains sugar, it might not contain *added sugars* such as sucrose or high-fructose corn syrup.

Let's look at milk as an example: you read the label and see that it has 5 grams of sugar, but there are *no added sugars* in the ingredients list, which means the sugars in the milk occur naturally, making it acceptable for Cycle One. An exception is fruit juice; although it comes from a natural source—fruit—that source has been stripped of its healthy fiber and thus has an extremely high fructose content.

This cycle is geared toward independence. Not only am I trying to free you from the health-sabotaging bonds of sugar, but also I'm trying to help you get free of your dependency on certain foods or behaviors. Once you learn to read labels and to shop wisely for yourself, the cycle will go much more smoothly and you'll be equipped with the tools to last you a lifetime.

As I tell my clients, "Learn the cycle to live the cycle!"

Sugar by Any Other Name

Many diets recommend a "weaning off" or "phasing out" period, where "treats" are allowed, if only in moderation. This goes against one of the central philosophies of habit alteration. It usually takes two to three weeks of total absence of a certain food to develop a sensitivity to it, so I do not allow a "free day" or "food pass" during a cycle until after clients have passed a habit test (see the end of this chapter for an example). I'm confident you can stick to this because you are eliminating only one negative dietary habit at a time.

In Cycle One, I'm not saying cut out milk or vegetables that have a sugar effect (like potatoes); I'm saying cut out **sugar**. By compartmentalizing one bad habit at a time, we can better control it and, eventually, eliminate it.

Avoid foods containing these sugars during Cycle One:

Corn syrups (also known as glucose syrup) —

Syrup made from corn starch and composed mainly of glucose. A series of chemical reactions are used to convert corn starch to corn syrup. It is a refined, unnatural sweetener.

Fructose—

Also known as levulose and fruit sugar, fructose is the sweetest of all the simple sugars. Fruits contain between 1 and 7% fructose, although some fruits have much higher amounts. This simple sugar is allowed to be consumed only where it is found naturally in fruit. No fruit juice of any kind is allowed in this cycle.

Fruit Concentrate/Sweetener—

This is what is lurking in many commercial juices. Since no juice of any kind is allowed in Cycle One, you probably won't come across it, but this is a fair warning to be on the lookout! It contains 90 to 96% simple sugars like glucose. It is frequently used in jellies.

Granulated Cane Juice—

Made from organically grown sugar cane juice that has been processed and dehydrated. It's a simple sugar that tastes much like brown sugar. It is 96% sucrose.

High-fructose corn syrups (HFCS) —

A modified form of corn syrup that has an increased level of fructose. There has been an effort by the corn industry to push the idea that HFCS is the same as regular sugar (which would be detrimental enough) but, unfortunately, scientific evidence proves this not to be true. In a comparative study conducted by a Princeton University research team using two groups of rats, one of which was fed water sweetened with HFCS and the other fed water sweetened with plain table sugar, results showed that the rats fed HFCS gained significantly more weight than did the rats fed table sugar (Servan-Schrieber 2010).

> Male rats in particular ballooned in size: Animals with access to high-fructose corn syrup gained 48 percent more weight than those eating a normal diet. In humans, this would be equivalent to a 200-pound man gaining 96 pounds. "These rats aren't just getting fat; they're demonstrating characteristics of obesity, including substantial increases in abdominal fat and circulating triglycerides," said Princeton graduate student Miriam Bocarsly. "In humans, these same characteristics are known risk factors for high blood pressure, coronary artery disease, cancer and diabetes."
>
> Dr. Servan-Schreiber explains the science behind it like this: High-fructose corn syrup and sucrose are both compounds that contain the simple sugars fructose and glucose, but there are at least two clear differences between them. First, sucrose is composed of equal amounts of the two simple sugars—it is 50 percent fructose and 50 percent glucose—but the typical high-fructose corn syrup used in this study features a slightly imbalanced ratio, containing 55 percent fructose and 42 percent glucose. Larger sugar

molecules called higher saccharides make up the remaining 3 percent of the sweetener. Second, as a result of the manufacturing process for high-fructose corn syrup, the fructose molecules in the sweetener are free and unbound, ready for absorption and utilization. In contrast, every fructose molecule in sucrose that comes from cane sugar or beet sugar is bound to a corresponding glucose molecule and must go through an extra metabolic step before it can be utilized.

Long story short, avoid high-fructose corn syrup!

Honey—

Honey is a mixture of sugars. It contains glucose, fructose, and sucrose. Although natural and containing antioxidants, it is not allowed in Cycle One because research shows that it can retard the habit-altering process and prevent your body from developing a sensitivity to concentrated sugars.

Maple Syrup—

A distinctive, delicious syrup made from the sap of sugar maple and black maple trees. It takes about five gallons of sap to produce a pint of syrup that is 65% sucrose and 35% water, and which contains a minute quantity of minerals.

Sucrose (table sugar, white or brown; made from either sugar cane or sugar beets)—

Sugar has been linked to weight gain, reduced immune function, and diseases such as diabetes. It has also been proven to leach minerals and vitamins from the body, making it an anti-nutrient. It is absolutely not allowed in Cycle One.

Trace Amounts of Sugar

You may encounter some products that contain some of these ingredients but still say zero sugars. By law, the U.S. Food and Drug Administration (FDA) allows any food that has 0.5 grams of sugar or less to be called sugar-free. They basically round down. There are also certain foods that contain 1 or 2 grams of sugar, such as non-dairy whipped topping or regular Cheerios. This amount of sugar is negligible and will not retard the habit-forming process. Don't go above 2 grams, at which point it can no longer be considered only a trace amount.

You will also run into many types of bread that contain small amounts of sugar. You can avoid them by choosing one of the many low-carb options, but don't go crazy trying to avoid bread. Our research suggests that cutting out high-sugar foods is effective for building sensitivity to sugars. The amount of sugar (in the form of sucrose or corn syrup) used even in white breads is small enough that it won't retard the habit-altering process. Breads with minimal traces of sugars are allowed in Cycle One. *However, do not eat sweet dessert breads or breads with honey.* This *will* disrupt the habit-altering process. Bottom line, if any bread tastes sweet, do not eat it.

Review of Acceptable Sweeteners

Despite what you may have heard, dozens of studies support the safety of artificial sweeteners in moderation. According to the National Cancer Institute, FDA-approved sweeteners have not demonstrated clear evidence of an association with cancer in humans (NCI 2009).

Let's review most of the popular artificial sweeteners and a brief history of each. Since this is a highly debated topic, I'll leave it to your best judgment which sweetener to choose, but I recommend sticking with the Stevia and Stevia blends because of their added health benefits. All of the sweeteners listed below are allowed in Cycle One.

Stevia (common name brands are Truvia, SweetLeaf, Steviva) —

In their natural state, Stevia leaves—which may be dried and crushed to a powder—are said to be 10–15 times sweeter than table sugar. The refined extract is, however, 200–300 times sweeter than sugar. Its medicinal uses include regulating blood sugar and preventing hypertension and tooth decay. Other studies show that it is a natural antibacterial and antiviral agent as well (Das et al. 2009). Stevia is actually very good for you! It is calorie- and carbohydrate-free. Stevia is a great sugar alternative for diabetics, those watching their weight, and anyone interested in maintaining their health.

Stevia blends (common name brand is Steviva Blend) —

A combination of stevia and erythritol—a sugar alcohol that exists naturally in many foods such as cheese, wine, watermelon, and mushrooms as well as in the bodies of both humans and animals. Erithrytol offers 70% of the sweetness of sucrose, so it could be an ideal sweetener alone but is commonly blended with other sweeteners. The combination of erythritol and stevia creates crystallization similar to that of sugar and has sweetness that measures cup-for-cup to sugar. Combining erythritol masks stevia's bitter flavor, which can be tasted if you use too much. The cup-for-cup measuring makes it very convenient when cooking or baking. Stevia and Stevia blends are the sugar substitute of choice for the Healthy Habit Plan. Since they can be hard to find and expensive, however, I recommend other options as well.

Acesulfame-k (also listed as Acesulfame-potassium; common name brands are Sunett, Sweet and Safe, Sweet One) —

200 times sweeter than sucrose (table sugar). The FDA approved it in 1988 as a general-purpose sweetener.

Aspartame (common brands are Equal, NutraSweet, SugarTwin) —

Up to 220 times sweeter than sucrose (table sugar). In 1996, the FDA approved aspartame in all foods and beverages. Aspartame is approved in more than 100 other countries. One gram of aspartame does contain 4 calories, but the amount required to sweeten foods is so minimal that it usually adds no calories per serving. The FDA has received complaints about possible side effects from aspartame; however, intense investigations by the Centers for Disease Control and Prevention (CDC) do not link those side effects to this artificial sweetener.

Saccharin (common name brands are Necta Sweet, Sweet 'N Low, Sweet 'N Low Brown) —

Up to 700 times sweeter than sucrose (table sugar). Saccharin is approved for use in the United States and 100 other countries. It contains 0 calories per gram and can be used for baking. Saccharin is commonly found in gum, prescription drugs, and cosmetics. The FDA proposed a ban on Saccharin in 1977 after early studies indicated that it caused cancer in lab rats. All products that contained saccharin were forced to carry a warning label. Later studies by the FDA as well as by the National Cancer Institute failed to link it to any form of cancer in humans. Thus the warning label requirements were retracted in 2000 (NCI 2009).

Sucralose (common name brand is Splenda) —

Sweetening power of this artificial sweetener is 600 times that of sucrose (table sugar). It was approved by the FDA, the European Union, and various individual countries in 1999. It is the only artificial sweetener made from sugar. It contains zero calories per gram and can be used for baking.

A Brief Description of Sugar Alcohols

Sugar alcohol is neither "sugar" nor "alcohol." Sugar alcohols, also known as *polyols,* are commonly used as sweeteners in many sugar-free products. Unlike artificial sweeteners, sugar alcohol occurs naturally and comes from many plant products.

> **Habit Helper—**
>
> *Sugar alcohols provide fewer calories and have little effect on blood sugar levels. Because of this dual effect, they are allowed in Cycle One to help wean you off "real" concentrated sweeteners.*

Sugar alcohols are low in calories, do not cause tooth decay, and have little effect on blood sugar levels. They are allowed in Cycle One to help wean you off "real," concentrated sweeteners. They are commonly found in low-carb products. Consuming too much can cause bloating or have a laxative effect (except for erythritol), so be careful not to overuse them. Here is a list of some of the most common sugar alcohols.

Erythritol—

As mentioned above, this sweetener exists naturally in many foods such as cheese, wine, watermelon, and mushrooms. It is also present in the bodily fluids of humans and animals. It offers 70% of the sweetness of sucrose, so it makes an ideal sweetener alone but is commonly blended with other sweeteners.

Isomalt—

A natural sugar alcohol produced from beets that is approximately 45 to 60% as sweet as sugar. Commonly found in hard candies and cough drops.

Mannitol—

Occurs naturally in sweet potatoes, carrots, pineapples, and other fruits and vegetables; about 50% relative sweetness of sugar.

Sorbitol—

Found naturally in vegetables and some fruit and only about 60% as sweet as sugar. It is often found in chewing gums and hard candies.

Xylitol—

Is also called "wood sugar" and occurs naturally in fruits, vegetables, mushrooms, and corncobs. It has very nearly the same sweetness as sugar (sucrose). It has also been proven to prevent tooth decay and is commonly found in chewing gums.

Proceed with Caution—
Foods to Watch Out for in Cycle One

The more you begin to monitor what you put into your mouth—and how it affects your body—the more you will notice the very obvious responses that some foods create as compared with others. You can probably do so already. For instance, a slice of pizza probably makes you feel one way while an order of broccoli makes you feel another. Both physically and emotionally, an apple has one effect on your body; an ice cream cone has another.

The foods listed below creep into a gray area that many of us ignore as we make poor eating choices. For instance, for decades yogurt has been seen as the ultimate dietary food, but did you know it can often be high in sugar? Salads are another diet staple, but depending on the dressing you use, that salad could derail a day's otherwise low sugar intake.

To help steer you through this area, here is a list of commonly overlooked foods to avoid during Cycle One because of their high (hidden) sugar content.

BBQ sauces

Certain salad dressings

Colas

Corn syrups

Frozen foods with high sugar content

Gum

Honey

Jellies

Juices of any kind

Ketchup

Maple syrup

Molasses

Sugar-added breakfast cereals

Syrups

Yogurt (except plain or artificially sweetened)

Fight Your Cravings with These Seven Sweet Treats

Symptoms of sugar withdrawal, such as mood swings, cravings for sugary foods, and lower energy, are strongest in the first week. Use these items to put out those sugar-craving fires.

Sugar-free hot chocolate (Swiss Miss, Nestle, or others)

Sugar-free jellies (Smuckers, for example)

Sugar-free popsicles

Sugar-free chocolate (Hershey's, Sorbee, and Whitman's all have sugar-free products. You can find others online at sugarlessshop.com, chocoholicsheaven.com, and lowcarbdiets.com to name a few. The sugarless shop has a sugar-free brownie mix that makes fantastic brownies.)

Sugar-free gum

Sugar-free ice cream

Fresh fruit

The first week will be the toughest of Cycle One, and these foods may not taste as good to you as the full-sugar versions but, if you stay consistent, all these items will start tasting more and more normal and eventually they will taste just like the "real" thing. For many of us, they are better than the "real" thing; or better said, they *are* the real thing!

If you're motivated and interested enough to go for it, then I know you can hang in there for about a week. Most people's taste buds will adapt quickly, but that doesn't mean you're ready to move on to the next cycle. NO! You need to remain on schedule; six weeks of eating concentrated sweetener-free choices. Your body will never enjoy sugar in the same way again if you make it through this cycle.

Cycle One Nutrition—
Frequently Asked Questions

1. **May I have honey, maple syrup or molasses during this cycle?**

   No. Although honey and molasses are both natural sweeteners that often contain traces of healthy vitamins and minerals, they are also very high in calories and sugars. For example, over 96% of the dry matter in honey is simple sugars: glucose, fructose, and even a little sucrose. It is higher in calories than regular white sugar! Grades A and B maple syrup are also very high in sucrose. If I allowed these natural sweeteners in the Healthy Habit Plan program, your initial sugar withdrawal would likely cause you to consume them in great quantities and prevent you from developing any sensitivity to concentrated sugar.

   You are welcome to eat these items once a week *after Cycle One* because, at that point, your body's newly developed sensitivity to sugar will protect you from going overboard.

   In moderation, I'm sure natural sweeteners are a healthier alternative when compared with regular sugars, considering the vitamins and minerals in many of them, but you probably won't crave them as much after this cycle. A word of caution: Be careful going straight for any concentrated sweetener after six weeks of being sugar free. By then your body will be very sensitive and may have a stronger reaction than you might expect.

2. **Isn't sugar natural? If so, why do you think it's so unhealthy?**

No. Sugar is only natural in its complete form, which is not the white granules you find at the store. Chewing on whole sugar cane would be significantly healthier because the fiber in the stalk is Mother Nature's way of protecting you. Sucrose lacks minerals and vitamins, and it must draw upon the body's micronutrient stores in order to be properly metabolized in the system. Refined table sugar is an anti-nutrient that causes many health problems.

3. **Why do you allow artificial sweeteners in your book? Aren't these items unnatural and unhealthy chemicals?**

I will not preach to you on why I think artificial sweeteners are safe. I will offer what I have experienced in my own life and seen in the lives of my clients. I have witnessed countless lives changed for the better when people replaced sugar with artificial sweeteners.

Artificial sweeteners are calorie free, have little to no impact on blood sugar levels, and will not cause weight gain. Sugar, on the other hand, *has* been linked to weight gain, reduced immune function, and diseases such as diabetes. It has also been proven to leach minerals and vitamins from the body (Appleton 2010).

You don't have to agree with me; again, I just share my thoroughly considered opinion and observations. This debate is not new; people have been arguing the health benefits (or risks) of artificial sweeteners since their creation. The reason I recommend using artificial sweeteners in the very first cycle is because doing so can lead to direct results, which is important for building confidence and consistency when following the Healthy Habit Plan. Artificial sweeteners are also readily available, making the switch as easy as possible.

4.   May I have milk?

Yes. The sugar in milk, called "lactose," is composed of one molecule of glucose and one of galactose. Because of the galactose content in milk, it is absorbed at a much slower rate into the blood stream, which means it doesn't disrupt blood sugar levels. This is a natural sugar found in dairy products, and it won't hurt you unless, of course, you are lactose intolerant! (This means you lack enough of the enzyme *lactase* that is required to break down the sugars and allow for proper absorption.) If you are lactose intolerant, milk might make you sick. Other than that, the calcium in dairy products has been proven to aid in weight loss, so it would be a mistake not to include at least some in your diet.

5.   Since artificial sweeteners are much sweeter than regular sugar, will I still crave sweet things?

Yes, in a sense. Even though artificial sweeteners taste much sweeter than sugar, the flavor is different, and the amounts you are using are less, which makes the sweetness similar to sugar. Even though it takes time to adapt your taste buds to artificial sweeteners, when you finally do, you will find that regular sugar has a much different taste and texture than it did before. The taste differs from person to person, but most describe regular sugar as tasting "heavy," with an almost "syrupy" sensation.

Of course, I haven't even addressed the spikes in blood sugar levels, depression, poor concentration, and anxiety that have all been linked to heavy sugar consumption. When you have negative reactions like this, your mind will start to associate these bad feelings with sugar and this in itself will decrease cravings. To finish answering your question, understand that getting on the Healthy Habit Plan will not eliminate your sweet tooth and was not designed to do so.

Contrary to popular belief, the sweet tooth is a very natural thing in humans. Before today's sugar overload, our sweet tooth actually aided in our health. Back in the pre-Twinkie days, people ate fresh fruits full of fiber, vitamins, minerals, and antioxidants.

Although fruit does contain sugar, people weren't consuming hundreds of pounds of refined sugars a year, which meant that strawberries and apples were as satisfying to them as a chocolate sundae is to us. Ideally, fruit makes the perfect dessert because the fiber prevents people from overdoing it, making it much harder to overindulge on apples, grapes, and bananas than on chocolate bars. Even though fruits are higher in calories than vegetables, they are an equally valuable part of our diet. Don't try to get rid of your sweet tooth—just refine it!

6. May I have alcohol?

Many alcohols are surprisingly low in sugars. Vodka, whiskey, gin, and tequila are all technically sugar and carbohydrate free. If you must drink, make sure there are no added sugars. Watch the mixes and syrups, and limit consumption to only once a week. Mixing these hard liquors with sugar-free fruit drinks or one of the popular low-carbohydrate drink mixes is technically allowed in Cycle One.

I say "technically," though, because alcohol of any kind can have a very damaging effect on your testosterone levels, the hormone responsible for muscle gain. Bottom line, alcohols are still damaging to your health, and I highly recommend you have only one drink, no more than once a week.

Many available studies tout the benefits of drinking wine, so you are allowed to consume up to half a glass of dry wine twice a week. Although technically a fermented juice, dry wines have extremely low sugar content.

The Healthy Habit Plan was never designed to remedy such damaging habits as drug or alcohol use, and if you feel you need to have more than one drink per week then you're not ready for the Healthy Habit Plan. It will do you no good trying to cut out sugar and saturated fat if you drink alcohol every night.

7. May I drink juice?

It is true that fructose, the simple sugar in fruit, is absorbed more slowly than other simple sugars because it has to be taken to the liver to be converted to glucose before it can be used. In addition, a benefit of eating the whole fruit is that it contains much-needed fiber. However, when you separate the fiber from the fructose (as in taking the juice from the fruit), it disrupts this process and allows the fructose in the juice to be more quickly absorbed.

So in this cycle, *juices are not allowed* and whole fruit is recommended for replacing it. Fructose accounts for a mere 5 to 7% of the nutrients in bananas, cherries, and apples, and even less for berries. Mother Nature knows the correct amount of this natural, but powerful, simple sugar you should be eating.

8. What about starches such as potatoes and bread?

Remember, this is not a carbohydrate reduction phase, so bread, pasta, potatoes, and rice are allowed. Right now we are focusing on the over-consumption of concentrated sugars that are often the basis for people's lack of health.

9. May I have a "free day" during the week to eat whatever I want?

In a word: NO! Although research suggests that people can develop sensitivities to sugars even by simply cutting sugar consumption in half, your sensitivity will not be nearly as strong. I have not limited you on anything else in this cycle, but it is crucial that you not cheat during this first cycle!

Instead, I want you to be so sensitive to any sugars by the end of this cycle that you can have only very, very small amounts! I want that can of regular soda to taste like pancake syrup. I want that ice cream sundae to taste horrible and give you a stomach ache. I want you to be so sensitive to sugars that an apple or orange will suffice for dessert!

This will not be possible if you eat small quantities of sweets during the week. If you do cheat, it will allow your bad habit to remain entrenched, and you will remain sugar free only to the extent of your willpower. Willpower does not last long term! Lifelong results are the goal in the Healthy Habit Plan, and you need well-established habits to accomplish that. *After Cycle One,* you will be allowed one free *meal* a week.

10. May I have sports drinks before my workout?

Some sports drinks contain lots of glucose, which is a simple sugar and is the most readily available form of energy for your body. Although it can improve performance, it is not ideal for weight loss. Many sports drinks also contain loads of sucrose and high-fructose corn syrup, which are not allowed in this cycle. Eat a piece of fruit and drink some water instead; our bodies were designed to obtain efficient energy from natural sources.

11. What if I eat at a restaurant or somewhere else away from my home?

This gets tricky. Order steak, fish, or chicken minus the rubs or sauces and eat a lot of veggies. Watch salad dressings and condiments. These days most restaurants already cater to the diabetic population and offer many sugar-free condiments. Likewise, if you're at a family celebration, make the best choices you can—focusing on simple proteins, vegetables, and fruits while steering away from those sugar-laden holiday goodies. If it's a potluck meal, all the better because you can bring items you know you can eat.

12. What about cereals?

Cereals that have no added sugars or high-fructose corn syrup are okay. Read the nutritional information and the ingredients list to know what you are putting in your body.

13. May I ever eat sugar again?

The real question is will you ever *want* to eat sugar again? The Healthy Habit Plan is not about willpower; it's about perfecting your habits so that your body will make definitive limits on how much bad food you can eat, if any. Natural sweeteners such as molasses, honey, or maple syrup would be preferable on your free meals *after Cycle One.* (Such sweeteners are easier on the gut simply because they're richer, sweeter, and people typically use less.)

However, if you feel like you just *have* to have a piece of real cake with real sugar, then indulging in a little treat once a week is alright, *but only after Cycle One*. By then, your new good habits will protect you from eating too much. If you do eat too much, it will happen only once and it will likely be a painful lesson for you.

You may even feel a little guilty—good! A little guilt keeps us in line.

14. **What's the best way to eat chocolate and still develop a habit or craving for fruit? I love chocolate!**

When you eat your fruit, use sugar-free chocolate sauce but reduce the overall amount after awhile. It's not that chocolate is bad for you, it's the sugar and fat that people put in the chocolate that are detrimental. Worry less about your chocolate habit but more about the kinds of chocolate you eat, meaning look for sugar-free varieties.

Cycle One Nutrition Habit Test

Habit, if not resisted, soon becomes necessity.

—St. Augustine

The Habit Test is something that makes this book unique. It is important that you do not move ahead in the cycles until you are certain that you have developed truly negative reactions to your once-favorite, but unhealthy, foods. Although you have been using motivation to help get you through this cycle, it is now time to allow your newly established habits to take over. People often have no idea how great an impact the foods they consume have on how they feel physically and mentally.

To take the test, you are to consume a large portion of the food you have been avoiding. A good test after Cycle One would be to eat a banana split. The point here is to gauge your reaction—the stronger the reaction, the stronger the developed habit.

This test can, and probably will, make you uncomfortable, but I feel it is necessary to ensure that in future cycles you will not be relying on willpower alone as you move forward. After you consume your forbidden food, I want you to wait about thirty to forty-five minutes before answering the questions below. It is critical that you answer honestly because your outcome will determine whether you are ready to move on to the next cycle.

1. *Did you enjoy the taste of your forbidden food?*
   A. Yes, I loved it and missed it. (1 point)
   B. No, it tasted too sweet and was horrible. (3 points)
   C. It was alright, but not what I remember. (2 points)

2. *Did you have any mild stomach aches or cramps?*
   A. No, not at all. (1 point)
   B. Yes, I did experience a little stomach pain. (3 points)
   C. A little discomfort, but not much. (2 points)

3. *Did you have severe reactions such as diarrhea or vomiting?*
   A. I felt bad, but did not get sick. (2 points)
   B. Yes, I threw up (or got diarrhea). (3 points)
   C. I experienced no severe side effects. (1 point)

4. *Did you really crave your forbidden food?*
   A. No, not at all. (3 points)
   B. Yes, I really looked forward to my forbidden food. (1 point)
   C. A little, but not as much as I used to. (2 points)

5. *Did you experience any lethargy?*
    A. Yes, a lot. (3 points)
    B. No, not at all. (1 point)
    C. A little, but not much. (2 points)

6. *Did you experience unusual chest pressure after the consumption of your forbidden food?*
    A. Some, but not much. (2 points)
    B. Yes, a lot. (3 points)
    C. No, not at all. (1 point)

7. *Did you feel depressed after the consumption of your forbidden food?*
    A. Yes, I did feel depressed. (3 points)
    B. No, not at all. (1 point)
    C. I felt a little down, but not much. (2 points)

8. *Did you feel sudden restlessness or anxiety after the consumption of your forbidden food?*
    A. Yes, I did. (3 points)
    B. No, not at all. (1 point)
    C. I felt a little anxiety, but not much. (2 points)

9. *Did you feel cranky or moody after your forbidden food?*
    A. A bit, but not much. (2 points)
    B. Yes, very cranky. (3 points)
    C. No, I was in a great mood. (1 point)

10. *Did you even want to splurge today?*
    A. Yes, a lot. (1 point)
    B. No, not at all. (3 points)
    C. A little, but not much. (2 points)

Scoring Your Nutrition Test

If you scored 24 to 30, this is good news. It means you have developed a physical need to avoid the forbidden food. Not only have you developed a real sensitivity, but you have also lost your cravings and taste for it. To keep your sensitivity at high levels, please only have one free meal a week. You may not even crave it, but *do not overindulge* or you could experience very uncomfortable side effects.

If you scored 17 to 23, then you need to add another two weeks to your cycle. This is not a bad thing; it just means that your body is trying to hold on to some of its old habits. It's not unusual for people to need to extend the cycle for a couple of weeks. This score still means you have at least *started* to experience some negative reactions to concentrated sugars, so you're heading in the right direction.

If you scored 10 to 16, you need to find out if the forbidden food is sneaking into your diet somewhere, intentionally or not. When you get a score this low it means your body is having trouble building sensitivity. Don't get frustrated, you just need to take a look at your diet and really see if there is anything that could be disrupting the habit-altering process. What you need to do is add three weeks to Cycle One and then take the test again. After that, you should at least score in the 17-to-23 range. Don't cheat! Consistency is the key.

Cycle One Fitness

To Do—

- *Start being active every day by focusing on activities and chores that need to be done anyway.*

Much as the nutrition aspect of Cycle One focuses on eliminating just one ingredient—sugar—from your diet, the exercise arm of the first cycle is also intended as a "get your feet wet" phase, so that you have the time and energy to accomplish your fitness goals on your own terms and in your own time.

In this cycle, you will concentrate on Level 1 activities. These include lawn mowing, cleaning, dog walking, or any general labor activity. My clients always love that the chores they have to do anyway count as a part of the Cycle One program. Outside of this, the only other form of exercise that is allowed is easygoing group training or maybe brisk walking with your spouse or partner. These activities are to be done every day for twenty to thirty minutes at a time.

If you have worked out for awhile and feel this is not enough, then I will give you permission to jump ahead to Level 2 exercises, but *not* to skip the dietary guidelines. This is the only cycle in which I allow you to jump ahead. For most people, I strongly recommend you go in order and ease into an active lifestyle.

> ### Habit Helper—
>
> *Most people brush their teeth every day because good oral hygiene takes daily maintenance. The same is true for your physical health. Exercising for a minimum of 30 minutes every day at varying levels of intensity is the best way to reach and maintain a healthy level of fitness, not to mention making it easier to develop a habit for doing so. Find a creative way to stay active. Soon enough, you'll be looking forward to your daily exercise!*

Level 1 Activities

Make sure that you are not only serious about the activities you choose but also mindful of how it feels to do them. For some of you, this may be your first time exercising in years, maybe even ever. For others, this might seem like I'm telling you to walk instead of run, but stick with it.

When you truly learn to enjoy Level 1 Activities and do them like you're enjoying them, the time will fly by, and you'll want to do them more often—and for longer periods of time. Examples of allowed activities are:

Dog walking—

Great exercise if you move fast. Move quickly and do it for at least 20 minutes for a great Level 1 Activity.

House cleaning—

Moving fast throughout a house scrubbing, vacuuming, and cleaning will get your heart rate up. Try jogging in between rooms.

Lawn mowing—

Great aerobic exercise if it's done with a push lawn mower; it really works the legs. Please be careful of the heat in summer, especially if you live in a hot part of the country. Drink lots of water and, if possible, mow during the morning hours.

Car washing—

When I say wash a car, I mean *scrub* it and try to get it as clean as possible by hand. It can be a great workout. Want more? Wax your car by hand. Other household activities, like wood chopping, gardening, snow shoveling, and building, can be great Level 1 exercises.

Note: Make it a habit to park far from a store and walk in. Also, take the stairs when possible and when it's safe—pretend there's no such thing as elevators.

Activities Not Allowed

Remember, we are in Cycle One, not Cycle Four. Don't skip ahead because you think I'm holding you back. The beauty of these cycles is that they're very precise, and they're very personal. Within those 20 to 30 minutes for each Level 1

> ### Habit Helper—
>
> *When you start to enjoy Level 1 activities, the time will fly by, and you'll want to do them more often and for longer periods of time. Go for it!!*

Activity, you can put as much or as little gusto in as you like. At first, it might be hard to get excited about doing housework or mowing the lawn, but as your body gets used to this level of activity every day it will start to crave it, and then you will start to look forward to it, putting more effort into it for longer periods of time.

For best results, stick to the guidelines and follow the rules. To that end, here are some activities *not* to do during Cycle One.

Solo gym workouts—

It takes tremendous motivational fuel to drive to the gym and make yourself get on a treadmill or lift weights. With no supervision, it's easy to breeze through it with little intensity, or to plan to do it and then not show up at all. Rather than either of these scenarios, I want you to avoid the gym during your six weeks of Cycle One.

Home workouts—

Doing classic home workouts, whether using exercise DVDs or

machines, requires tremendous motivation to get up off the couch. Working out at home is the worst way for a beginner to develop a fitness habit, because there are too many distractions: chores, bills, kids, TV, and more. That's why so many well-intentioned people end up using their home-workout equipment as clothing racks. Instead of trying and failing to work out at home, I want you to avoid it for Cycle One.

High-intensity advanced workouts of any kind—

These are not allowed in this cycle! Remember, baby steps!

Cycle One Fitness—
Frequently Asked Questions

1. **What if this is not enough exercise for me? I want more!**

    It's surprisingly common for many people to already have a basic need for exercise. In this case, you are allowed moderate group training classes such as toning, weight training, aerobics, and spinning. These classical workouts are great as long as you do them in a group setting. Don't attempt to do classical workouts alone, and don't yet try *advanced* group training classes. In other words, you can move to Cycle Two Fitness but no further.

2. **Is playing a sport consistently allowed in Cycle One?**

    I suggest you move to the Level 2 activities. Do not move to Level 2 dietary guidelines, just exercise. This cycle allows you to participate in motivational sports and hobbies and is the only cycle in which you are allowed to move ahead.

3. Is gardening really enough exercise if that's all I do?

No, but I'm not looking to overwhelm you with a too-rigorous exercise program at this stage. I am trying to get your mind and body to *slowly* develop a need for activity. In this case, consistency is more important than the specific activity. Pay attention to your heart rate while you garden. Are you just pulling weeds crouched in the same position for twenty minutes, or are you raking leaves? Listen to your body. If you know you're not getting in the right level of activity when you garden, add a brisk walk to your day. And don't worry too much; more intense activities will be required in future cycles. By then, though, you will probably *want* to do more.

4. What if I want to lift weights?

Do the mild group training classes that use weights. In Cycle Three you will be allowed to hire a trainer if you want more intense weight lifting. Understand that this sport takes tremendous willpower and discipline to be done consistently because there is typically a fairly strong level of physical discomfort. I generally don't recommend weight-training programs (especially done alone) for those with no need for intense levels of exercise yet.

5. What if I live in an apartment and don't have many chores to do?

There are always things you can do. Remember, this is more of a philosophy than a set diet or exercise routine. If you live in a big city, walk ten blocks instead of taking a taxi, or take the stairs to your apartment instead of riding the elevator.

Go dancing. Take up yoga or another popular group training class. Get a hyperactive dog. Give your neighbors a break and walk their dogs or run around the park with their kids. Volunteer in busy soup kitchens or community beautification programs. Be creative! Find things that you either have to do or really enjoy doing.

Cycle One Exercise Habit Test

You will take this Exercise Habit Test on the same day as your Nutrition Habit Test. You are to be extremely inactive that day, and at the end of the day take the test below. Answer the questions truthfully about how you felt during your sedentary day.

Be honest, because your score will determine whether or not you are ready to move forward. The goal is to establish a physical need to be active every day because well-established habits can last a lifetime.

Sleep is equally important. Make sure you are getting seven to eight hours of sleep a night. If not, all the exercise and nutrition in the world will do little to make you feel better.

1. *Did you feel lethargic today?*
   A. Yes, I did. (3 points)
   B. No, not at all. (1 point)
   C. A little, but not much. (2 points)

2. *Did you feel anxious or nervous today?*
   A. No, not at all. (1 point)
   B. A little, but it didn't bother me. (2 points)
   C. Yes, I did. (3 points)

3. *How was your concentration level?*

A. I was a little scatterbrained today, but not a whole lot. (2 points)

B. My concentration level was horrible. (3 points)

C. It was perfectly fine. (1 point)

4. *Did you feel guilty for being so inactive?*
   A. Yes, I felt very guilty. (3 points)
   B. No, not at all. (1 point)
   C. A little. (2 points)

5. *Did you feel hungrier than usual?*
   A. No, not at all. (3 points)
   B. Yes, a lot. (1 points)
   C. A little bit. (2 points)

6. *Did you really want to get up and do something active?*
   A. Yes, I did. (3 points)
   B. I could have gone either way. (2 points)
   C. No, I enjoyed lying around all day. (1 point)

Scoring Your Exercise Test

If you scored 15 to 18, then congratulations; you are becoming habitually healthy. Your mind and body now need activity. Soon, you will become more and more "addicted" to physical activity with more intensity. More intensity means more muscle, more burned calories, and an athletic body.

If you scored 10 to 14, then you're heading in the right direction. Don't get frustrated! Everyone develops habits at a different pace. Many things, like past activity experience, genetics, diet, and more, play a part in your overall fitness level, as well as how quickly you adapt to physical change. Don't be in a hurry. Stay with this cycle for another two weeks and then take the test again.

If you scored 6 to 9, then something is interfering with the habit-altering process. Before you get frustrated, honestly answer these questions:

- *Are you following the activity guidelines exactly?*

  If not, then you are probably burning yourself out. Remember, advanced workout programs require a real habit for exercise in order to be consistent. Anyone can work out hard for a week, but you've got a bigger prize in mind—habits. *Slow way down!*

- *Are you consistent with your activity requirements?*

  Just like the diet section, for a habit to be established, consistency is everything. Some people like the concept of the Healthy Habit Plan but are not motivated enough to wholeheartedly pursue it. Unfortunately, where there is no motivation, there is no real consistency. If you're having trouble being consistent, make sure you are moving slowly and doing activities you enjoy.

- *Are you eating properly?*

  Make sure you are following the nutrition guidelines perfectly as you move through your cycles. If you are developing a habit for intense physical activity while leaving your eating habits untouched, then this is counterproductive. The more active you are, the higher quality food and energy your body will need.

If you answered "no" to any of the above questions, add three weeks to your current cycle and then try the test again. This does not mean you have failed; it just means your habit of being sedentary is fairly ingrained. Don't fret. It takes time to change your habits.

The only way to beat a habit is with another habit. This is exactly what we are trying to do but it takes time, and you may stumble a little along the way. Research proves that it takes most people four to five attempts to quit smoking but, as long as they keep trying, they eventually succeed. Develop a habit to never give up. This habit will do you much good in everything you pursue.

> **Habit Helper—**
>
> *Soon you will become more and more "addicted" to physical activity with more intensity. More intensity means more muscle, more burned calories, and a trimmer body.*

Chapter 6 References

Appleton, Nancy. 2010. "146 Reasons Why Sugar Is Ruining Your Health." rheumatic.org (accessed June 24, 2010).

Das, Kuntal, Raman Dang, and Nilesh Gupta. 2009. "Comparative Antimicrobial Potential of Different Extracts of Leaves of *Stevia rebaudiana* Bert." *International Journal of Natural Engineering Sciences* 3, no. 1: 59–69.

National Cancer Institute. 2009. "Artificial Sweeteners and Cancer." August 5. www.cancer.gov (accessed June 17, 2010).

Servan-Schreiber, David. 2010. "Scientific Evidence Supports the Dangers of High-Fructose Corn Syrup." *Anti-Cancer: A New Way of Life.* March 30. www.anticancerbook.com (accessed 2010).

7—Cycle Two

Habits are safer than rules; you don't have to watch them. And you don't have to keep them, either; they keep you.   —Dr. Frank Crane

Cycle Two Nutrition: Healthier Carbohydrates

To Do—

- *Begin consuming carbs in a healthier ratio with vegetables and proteins.*

- *Switch all refined carbs to healthier, whole grain versions.*

- *Maintain Cycle One sugar requirements.*

This is a six-week cycle, divided into two parts that are each three weeks in length. The goal in the first phase of Cycle Two is to develop a habit of eating carbohydrates in more balanced proportions. After this, we will move on to the next phase in which you will develop an overall taste for healthier carbs, such as whole grains.

Carbohydrate Mixing

In this phase, you are allowed to eat any starch or carbohydrate whether it's pasta, bread, potatoes, and so forth, as long as it's *physically* combined with an equal amount of vegetables and/or protein. I do not mean just a balanced meal in which you can eat the pasta and pick around the veggies. I mean you have to literally stir it up and eat it all together (think Chinese food or stew). For example, if you want to eat a cup of pasta or rice make sure you combine it with an equal or greater part of vegetables and protein. If you want bread then have a sandwich with a ton of veggies and meat. If you want chips, crush them up in chili or chunky salsa. This method has proven to be very effective in altering taste buds and developing a taste for high-fiber fruit and, more important, vegetables (a crucial part of any diet) and in beginning to develop a habit for balanced meals.

Most people don't eat many vegetables, and just telling them that vegetables are good for them doesn't always work. Less than 5% of the population have a fruit and a vegetable every day. People may put them on their plate but then just pick around them and go back for more pasta.

When you physically mix your starches with vegetables, it will make the vegetables more enjoyable. It's also portion control in disguise because you're not eating as much pasta as you normally would, allowing the protein and fiber from the meat and vegetables to fill you up more quickly, leaving less room for more carbs. Furthermore, when you re-acquaint your taste buds with vegetables, your body will eventually start to crave them.

So the rule is: Do not pick around the protein or the vegetables!

You have to eat meat and/or veggies whenever you eat starch. You may have to force yourself to eat certain vegetables in the beginning, but if you stay consistent, I promise that your body will learn to love them. I not only want you to develop a habit for healthy foods, but also I'm teaching your body to *need* balanced meals. This method works, and I think it is one of the best little techniques in the book.

Here are some examples of meals you can prepare:

- *Small bowl of no-sugar, high-fiber cereal with milk, plus two eggs*

- *Spaghetti with heavy meat and vegetable sauce* (Use equal amounts of sauce and pasta.)

- *Stews with vegetables, meat, and potatoes*

- *Sandwiches with meat and extra tomatoes, lettuce, cucumbers, pickles, and sprouts*

- *Soft taco with meat and extra vegetables*

- *Pasta salad with double vegetables and meat*

- *Chinese recipes* (Use sweeteners only once a week to maintain sugar sensitivity.)

- *Goulash with pasta, meat, and vegetables*

- *Plain pasta, vegetables, and chicken combined with a light, non-sweetened sauce*

- *Homemade hamburger with thin bun, meat patty, and loads of vegetables* (I use bread for the bun.)

- *Homemade chili mixed with meat, beans, and pasta or crackers*

- *Homemade tomato salsa mixed with crushed chips* (Eat quickly or chips get soft. Note: you can scoop the salsa as long as there is more salsa than chip with each scoop.)

- *Medium-sized potato stuffed with vegetables and meat*

- *Redskin potatoes and vegetables with side of meat*

- *Oatmeal with fruit plus two eggs* (Or, you can add a scoop of protein powder to the oatmeal.)

Switching to Whole Grain, Healthier Carbs

The second part of this cycle kicks in for the next three weeks. Switch to whole grain and/or healthier versions of pasta, chips, crackers, and breads.

- *White and wheat pasta have virtually the same glycemic rating (how fast it is broken down in the blood stream), and whole grain wheat has maybe 1 gram more fiber than does white pasta.*

  Pasta, whether white or wheat, will not hurt you if you combine it properly with each meal. In no way am I saying that white pasta is better for you than whole grain, but the difference is minimal. Egg noodles, however, have a significantly lower glycemic index as well as a pleasing texture. Furthermore, some pasta brands, such as "Smart Taste," have added protein to their pasta, making them a good choice as well. Whatever pasta you choose, make sure to balance it with protein and vegetables.

- *Go for the baked chips with zero trans fats.*

  Chips are okay as long as you treat them like a starch. Crush them in chili, chunky salsa, salads, on a sandwich (yes, really). Do not eat them alone. Crackers are to be consumed in the same manner as chips: in stews, chilis, soups, on salads, or with any meal that has a high vegetable and protein content. Treat them as your starch in the meal. Use the whole grain, no sugar, and low sodium versions such as Healthy Harvest brand crackers. If you want a second helping, you have to eat a second helping of every part of the meal.

- *Look for breads made from whole grain.*

  Now is the time to start being more particular about the quality of breads you consume. Since many wheat breads now available have no more fiber than their white counterparts, become a label reader and select breads based on their fiber content—the more fiber the better. Several "double fiber" breads are available and are great choices. Pacific Bakery and Ezekiel are even better breads since they have no sugar and a good amount of fiber. Also, avoid breads that have honey or sugar or high-fructose corn syrup in the ingredient list.

A Comment on Second Helpings and Additional Tips

If you want a second serving, you are welcome to have it—just try this technique first. Wait ten minutes, maybe have a breath mint or glass of water and then, if you're still hungry, go ahead and get seconds. Many times people eat so fast they don't realize that they're full. Mint has also been proven to reduce appetite. *Again, wait ten minutes before seconds.*

If it's suitable to your taste, try including several spicy dishes in your weekly meal plan. Studies have shown that spicy foods seem to suppress appetite.

Another technique is to drink two large glasses of water ten to fifteen minutes before your meal. This gives you a feeling of fullness so the amount you consume is less.

Cycle Two Nutrition—
Frequently Asked Questions

1. **Do I need to watch my fat intake?**

   No, the only thing I would highly recommend is to prepare most of your own meals. Don't use this concept with fast food. It simply does not work well because you can't be sure what they are putting in your food (in terms of sugars, additives, and extra fats).

2. **Do I *have* to mix? Can't I just eat a balanced meal?**

   If you can honestly get a cup of pasta, a cup of meat, and a cup of vegetables and eat them in that portion without skipping the veggies or going back for seconds on the pasta, then go for it. But watch how you do! If you catch yourself avoiding a food group, then I strongly recommend the mixing technique, especially if you're not used to eating balanced meals. This works!

3. **May I go back for a second serving?**

Yes, so long as you have equal parts of everything: meat, vegetables, and starches; but remember the ten-minute rule first.

4. When do we start counting calories?

You do not have to be a calorie counter in this cycle. Protein and fiber will give you a full feeling much quicker than a plate of pasta. You will find that as you start refining your dietary habits and eating healthier, well-balanced meals, you will not need as much food to feel full. But to answer your question, I address calorie counting in Cycle Four.

5. Do I have to add meat?

I would definitely recommend it, but if meat is not available or you're not in the mood for it, you can substitute beans. Beans have protein and fiber, but I would prefer you have a complete protein, such as meat. Consider adding tasteless protein cooking powders or eggs to properly balance your meals.

6. What if I don't eat meat?

There is a way to get all the essential amino acids from a vegetarian diet, but it involves combining many specific proteins in order to make a complete protein. I would highly recommend getting a book on preparing healthy vegetarian dishes. When you eat vegetarian the right way (not living on pasta, rice, and chips), it can be a very healthy diet. Most people don't have any idea how to prepare a truly vegetarian diet with properly balanced nutrients; it's not an easy path.

I'm not a personal fan of the vegetarian diet. My brother gave up being a vegetarian after almost twenty-one years of dedicated following. When he started eating meat again, he gained thirty pounds of muscle in a year and a half. His picture is on my website. This is only my opinion, and I have met many healthy vegetarians. With a little research, you should still be able to use the Healthy Habit Plan to help you go vegetarian. If you're not a vegetarian but are interested in being one, I recommend that you first go straight through, meat and all, and when you have developed real healthy habits, then apply the same approach to becoming vegetarian. The Healthy Habit Plan will be a good preliminary resource to help alter your unhealthy habits before taking on the strict vegetarian lifestyle. I assure you that despite what you may think, eliminating meat will do you no good if you can't break that chocolate cake habit.

7. **What other kinds of rice can I try in the second part of Cycle Two (Switching to Whole Grain, Healthier Carbs)?**

Anything but white, refined rice is acceptable.

8. **Can fruit be combined with starch?**

Yes and no. I allow you to combine starches and fruit only in the mornings to get fiber, vitamins, and minerals—such as with oatmeal and fruit, or whole wheat toast and fruit—as long as you have protein with it from milk, protein powder/shake, or eggs (my favorite). *Make sure you get some protein!* Fruit is higher in calories and sugar (natural sugar) than are vegetables, but vegetables have an equal amount (sometimes more) of vitamins, antioxidants, and minerals. You can eat small quantities of whole fruit as snacks in between your big meals or for dessert, but use veggies for the rest of your meals.

Cycle Two Recipes

CHICKEN AND RICE

8 drumsticks or thighs
1 cup long grain brown rice, uncooked
3 cups chicken stock
½ can condensed mushroom soup
1 medium onion, chopped
2 carrots, peeled and sliced
2 celery stalks, cleaned and sliced
¼ cup soy sauce
1 tsp ground pepper

Preheat oven to 350 degrees. Pull skin from chicken legs and discard. (This step is recommended for Cycle Two and required for Cycle Three.) In large bowl, stir together all remaining ingredients. Pour into large casserole dish. Add chicken and cover dish with lid or aluminum foil. Bake until chicken is completely cooked and all the liquid has been absorbed, 45 to 50 minutes. Serve using equal amounts of chicken and rice.

Stovetop Alternative: This recipe can also be prepared on the stovetop in a very large soup pot or dutch oven. Be sure to set heat on low to prevent burning. Keep lid on and no peeking until rice is tender, 45 to 50 minutes.

Makes approximately 4 to 6 servings

Spaghetti

1 lb ground beef
Olive oil to coat pan
4 cloves garlic, crushed
1 medium onion, diced
1 (7 oz) can sliced mushrooms, drained
¼ bell pepper, chopped
1 (28 oz) can whole tomatoes
1 (6 oz) can tomato paste
2½ Tbsp dried basil
2 Tbsp dried oregano
½ tsp dried thyme
½ tsp dried marjoram
½ tsp dried rosemary, crushed
1 tsp salt
½ tsp ground pepper
½ tsp crushed red pepper flakes (optional)
4 cups cooked pasta

Brown ground beef. Drain and rinse fat from meat and pan using hot water. (This step is recommended for Cycle Two and required for Cycle Three.) Place meat aside. Coat rinsed-out pan with olive oil, then add garlic, onion, mushrooms, and bell pepper. Sauté until onions are soft, about 3 minutes. Add canned tomatoes, crushing tomatoes by hand. Stir in tomato paste very thoroughly. Add all spices, stir well and let simmer on low for ten minutes, stirring occasionally. Add beef. Simmer for another ten minutes. Serve in equal amounts over pasta.

Makes about 4 servings

Feel free to freeze any remaining sauce for future use.

Pot Roast in a Slow Cooker

This recipe is designed for a very large slow cooker. Halve the recipe if using a smaller one.

3 Tbsp canola oil

1 medium rump roast (that can fit inside your slow cooker)

1 medium sweet or russet potato, peeled and cut into large pieces

4 carrots, peeled and cut into large pieces

1 large onion, peeled and quartered

3 celery stalks, cleaned and cut into large pieces

3 Tbsp all-purpose seasoning

Enough beef broth or water to cover meat and veggies in crock pot, about 2 to 3 cups

3 Tbsp cornstarch stirred into ¼ cup cold water

Salt and pepper to taste

Heat oil in large stainless steel skillet. Add roast and darkly brown on both sides. Place in slow cooker. Sprinkle with half the seasoning, salt, and pepper. Add all the vegetables and sprinkle with remaining seasoning. Add beef stock. Cook on low for 4 to 6 hours. Remove meat and vegetables from pot. Stir cornstarch mixture into broth and allow it to thicken for several minutes, stirring often. Cut meat into large chunks and serve with vegetables and gravy.

Makes 4 to 6 servings

To enjoy this recipe in Cycle Three, select a lower fat roast and cut away all visible fat.

Farmer's Breakfast

½ lb lean breakfast sausage, cooked and chopped
2 Tbsp canola oil
1 medium russet or red skin potato, scrubbed and diced
1 small onion, chopped
½ bell pepper, chopped
½ cup low-fat cheddar cheese (shredded)
6 eggs

In large nonstick skillet, cook breakfast sausage and set aside. In same skillet, heat oil and add potatoes. Cook on medium-high heat for about 8 minutes or until potatoes are almost done. Add onions and peppers. Cook for 4 minutes longer. Add breakfast sausage and cook for 1 more minute. Crack eggs in different spots over mixture in skillet. Reduce heat to low. Cook until eggs are done to your liking:

Scrambled: stir often. Turn off heat and add cheese. Stir one more time and serve.

Not scrambled: Keep heat on low, sprinkle cheese on top, cover and cook until eggs are done to your liking.

Makes 6 servings

Cycle Two Nutrition Habit Test

The Habit Test is something that makes this book unique. It is important that you do not move ahead in the cycles until you are certain that you have developed truly negative reactions to your once-favorite, but unhealthy, foods. Although you have been using motivation to help get you through this cycle, it is now time to allow your newly established habits to take over. People often have no idea how great an impact the foods they consume have on how they feel physically and mentally.

To take the test, you are to consume a large quantity of the food that you have been avoiding. A good test after Cycle Two would be to eat a bowl of pasta and nothing else. The point here is to gauge your reaction—the stronger the reaction, the stronger the developed habit.

This test can and probably will be uncomfortable but I feel it is necessary to ensure that you will not be relying on willpower alone as you move forward. After you consume your forbidden food, I want you to wait about thirty to forty-five minutes and then answer the questions below. It is critical that you answer honestly because your outcome will determine whether you are ready to move on to the next cycle.

1. *Did you enjoy the taste of your forbidden food?*
    A. Yes, I loved it and missed it. (1 point)
    B. No, it tasted horrible. (3 points)
    C. It was alright, but not what I remember. (2 points)

2. *Did you have any mild stomach aches or cramps?*
    A. No, not at all. (1 point)
    B. Yes, I did experience a little stomach pain. (3 points)
    C. A little discomfort, but not much. (2 points)

3. *Did you have severe reactions such as diarrhea or vomiting?*
    A. I felt bad, but did not get sick. (2 points)
    B. Yes, I threw up (or got diarrhea). (3 points)
    C. I experienced no severe side effects. (1 point)

4. *Did you really crave your forbidden food?*
    A. No, not at all. (3 points)
    B. Yes, I really looked forward to my forbidden food. (1 point)
    C. A little, but not as much as I used to. (2 points)

5. *Did you experience any lethargy?*
    A. Yes, a lot. (3 points)
    B. No, not at all. (1 point)
    C. A little, but not much. (2 points)

6. *Did you experience unusual chest pressure after the consumption of your forbidden food?*
    A. Some, but not much. (2 points)
    B. Yes, a lot. (3 points)
    C. No, not at all. (1 point)

7. *Did you feel depressed after the consumption of your forbidden food?*
    A. Yes, I did feel depressed. (3 points)
    B. No, not at all. (1 point)
    C. I felt a little down, but not much. (2 points)

8. *Did you feel sudden restlessness or anxiety after the consumption of your forbidden food?*
    A. Yes, I did. (3 points)
    B. No, not at all. (1 point)
    C. I felt a little anxiety, but not much. (2 points)

9. *Did you feel cranky or moody after your forbidden food?*
    A. A bit, but not much. (2 points)
    B. Yes, very cranky. (3 points)
    C. No, I was in a great mood. (1 point)

10. *Did you even want to splurge today?*
   A. Yes, a lot. (1 point)
   B. No, not at all. (3 points)
   C. A little, but not much. (2 points)

Scoring Your Nutrition Test

If you scored 24 to 30, this is good news. It means you have developed a physical need to avoid the forbidden food. Not only have you developed a real sensitivity, but you have also lost your cravings and taste for it. To keep your sensitivity at high levels, please have only one free meal a week. You may not even crave it, but *do not overindulge* or you could experience very uncomfortable side effects.

If you scored 17 to 23, then you need to add another two weeks to your cycle. This is not a bad thing; it just means that your body is trying to hold on to some of its old habits. It's not unusual for people to need to extend the cycle for a couple of weeks. This score still means you have at least *started* to experience some negative reactions to forbidden food, so you're heading in the right direction.

If you scored 10 to 16, you need to find out if the forbidden food is sneaking into your diet somewhere, intentionally or not. When you get a score this low it means your body is having trouble building sensitivity. Don't get frustrated, you just need to take a look at your diet and really see if there is anything that could be disrupting the habit-altering process. What you need to do is add three weeks to Cycle One and then take the test again. After that, you should at least score in the 17-to-23 range. Don't cheat! Consistency is the key.

Cycle Two Fitness

To Do—

- *Find a moderate-intensity group training class, sport, or hobby. To be done three times weekly.*

- *Maintain Cycle One activities.*

In this cycle, you will focus on extracurricular activities and sports or hobbies to get you in shape. One-on-one basketball with a friend, or racquetball, tennis, touch football on the weekends, and so forth. Get involved with walking or running clubs. Find a motivating aerobics instructor. Take up karate or another martial art. Go hiking, rock climbing, or play golf. Basically, build your exercise regimen on fun, competitive, and/or social activities. These "games" can definitely get you in great shape, and because they're fun and typically something you enjoy doing, you will do them more often, with more intensity, and most important, with more consistency. *Do not* yet attempt classic gym workouts, mindlessly walking on the treadmill, or pumping out triceps extensions. You're not ready for this yet but you will be. Remember, the only types of workouts that are allowed in a gym are group training classes. Hang in there. You're doing great!

Note: In the following Level 2 Activities section, you must participate in at least one Level 2 activity three times a week. Every other day, plug in the previous Level 1 activities. You must do something active every day. If you find yourself extremely tired after participating in Level 2 activities, reduce them to just twice a week. At this point in the Healthy Habit Plan, consistency is more important than intensity for building a physical and mental need for exercise.

Level 2 Activities

- *Martial Arts*

- *Moderate group training classes*

- *Any sport such as soccer, racquet-ball, tennis, or golf* (these may be more intense but are generally more enjoyable, making adherence easier)

- *Hiking*

- *Running with a running club or group*

> ### Habit Helper—
>
> *I know how important support is, so much so that the cycles themselves force you to surround yourself with it. Don't be afraid to get out of your comfort zone. Doing so places you in a realistic environment for change.*

Activities Not Allowed

- *Home workout programs* (will be allowed in Level 4)

- *Classic solo gym workouts* (will be allowed in Level 4)

- *Weight lifting with trainer* (will be allowed in Level 3)

- *High-intensity cardio programs* (will be allowed in Level 3)

I know this cycle is different from what you might have expected, but understand that 95% of people quit their fitness and diet programs very early on. It takes a tremendous amount of motivation and willpower to push yourself through a long, hard run or weight-training session. I have learned that for people to be truly consistent with classic gym workouts, one must already have a physical and mental need for exercise. For you right now, your need for exercise is too small, and you're currently having to rely on motivation for your fuel. Give it time. Remember, baby steps.

People e-mail me all the time telling me that weight lifting is a sport and that they love it! If you are one of those rare individuals who sincerely enjoys weight lifting and has experience doing it, then treat it like a sport and get on a sensible program. But I still strongly recommend against the classic gym workouts, especially if your past experiences with weight-training routines have not been consistent or successful. Weight training can be physically uncomfortable and is the most taxing on your motivational fuel. Consider group weight-training programs.

Cycle Two Fitness—
Frequently Asked Questions

1. May I workout with a friend and count that as a group?

Well, not necessarily! Studies do show that people are more likely to continue their exercise program with a friend or spouse (Gumper 2005). However, if your friend is in good shape and has already developed a need for exercise, their routine will most likely burn you out quickly. Or, if your friend has zero health habits and is as new to exercise as you are, you might both lose momentum. In that scenario, I would highly recommend group training classes or fun, sport-based activities for both of you at this point! Getting two habitually unhealthy people, instead of just one, and throwing them into a gym will not increase either one's chances for success. I will let you make your best judgment. If your friend is very experienced and has a proven track record of consistency, then they might have some tips to keep you motivated and on track. In this case it could work. You could give it a try, although be on the lookout for signs that you've been left in the dust because they mentally and physically need exercise and you don't yet!

2. **How do I include weight training in my Healthy Habit Plan Cycle Two if it's not allowed? I have heard that it is so important.**

I don't allow people to do traditional weight training yet. Solo weight-training programs require tremendous motivation especially if your only interest in weight training is just because so many experts are telling you how important it is for your health. They are right! Weight-bearing exercise is very important for your health, but you can get it elsewhere. Many hobbies and sports such as martial arts, hiking, and tennis are considered weight bearing and can build muscle, so don't think you have to lift weights. So although weight lifting may be able to get you in great shape, it requires tremendous discipline to be consistent in this activity because there are, quite frankly, moderate to high levels of physical discomfort involved. Still, if you're dying to pump iron, consider group weight-training classes where an instructor is telling you what to do, how to do it, and how many reps. This will save your motivation. In Cycle Three, you can up your weight training with a personal trainer.

3. **Can I really get an efficient workout playing sports?**

Yes, especially at Level 2, which includes activities required at least three times a week. Give it a try; I think you'll be surprised. Go out and play racquetball hard for 20 to 30 minutes and just see if you're not sweating like crazy. Or take a karate or boxing class and see if it's not challenging enough. Just make sure you pick an activity you enjoy.

4. **Do things like golf or gardening count as required activity?**

    Yes, but remember you have to participate in at least one Level 2 activity three times a week. Gardening and golf will be fine on other days.

Cycle Two Exercise Habit Test

You will take this Exercise Habit Test on the same day as your Nutrition Habit Test. You are to be extremely inactive that day, and at the end of the day take the test below. Answer the questions truthfully about how you felt during your sedentary day.

Be honest, because your score will determine whether or not you are ready to move forward. The goal is to establish a physical need to be active every day because well-established habits can last a lifetime.

Sleep is equally important. Make sure you are getting seven to eight hours of sleep a night. If not, all the exercise and nutrition in the world will do little to make you feel better.

1. *Did you feel lethargic today?*
    A. Yes, I did. (3 points)
    B. No, not at all. (1 point)
    C. A little, but not much. (2 points)

2. *Did you feel anxious or nervous today?*

    A. No, not at all. (1 point)

    B. A little, but it didn't bother me. (2 points)

    C. Yes, I did. (3 points)

3. *How was your concentration level?*

    A. I was a little scatterbrained today, but not a whole lot.
       (2 points)

    B. My concentration level was horrible. (3 points)

    C. It was perfectly fine. (1 point)

4. *Did you feel guilty for being so inactive?*

    A. Yes, I felt very guilty. (3 points)

    B. No, not at all. (1 point)

    C. A little. (2 points)

5. *Did you feel hungrier than usual?*

    A. No, not at all. (3 points)

    B. Yes, a lot. (1 point)

    C. A little bit. (2 points)

6. *Did you really want to get up and do something active?*

    A. Yes, I did. (3 points)

    B. I could have gone either way. (2 points)

    C. No, I enjoyed lying around all day. (1 point)

Scoring Your Exercise Test

If you scored 15 to 18, then congratulations; you are becoming habitually healthy. Your mind and body now need activity. Soon, you will become more and more "addicted" to physical activity with more intensity. More intensity means more muscle, more burned calories, and an athletic body.

If you scored 10 to 14, then you're heading in the right direction. Don't get frustrated! Everyone develops habits at a different pace. Many things, like past activity experience, genetics, diet, and more, play a part in your overall fitness level, as well as how quickly you adapt to physical change. Don't be in a hurry. Stay with this cycle for another two weeks and then take the test again.

If you scored 6 to 9, then something is interfering with the habit-altering process. Before you get frustrated, honestly answer these questions:

- *Are you following the activity guidelines exactly?*

  If not, then you are probably burning yourself out. Remember, advanced workout routines require a real habit for exercise in order to be consistent. Anyone can work out hard for a week, but you've got a bigger prize in mind—habits. *Slow way down!*

- *Are you consistent with your activity requirements?*

  Just like the diet section, for a habit to be established, con-sistency is everything. Some people like the concept of the Healthy Habit Plan but are not motivated enough to wholeheartedly pursue it. Unfortunately, where there is no motivation, there is no real consistency. If you're having trou-ble being consistent, make sure you are moving slowly and doing activities you enjoy.

- *Are you eating properly?*

  Make sure you are following the nutrition guidelines perfectly as you move through your cycles. If you are developing a habit for intense physical activity while leaving your eating habits untouched, then this is counterproductive. The more active you are, the higher quality food and energy your body will need.

If you answered "no" to any of the above questions, add three weeks to your current cycle and then try the test again. This does not mean you have failed; it just means your habit of being sedentary is fairly ingrained. Don't fret. It takes time to change your habits.

The only way to beat a habit is with another habit. This is exactly what we are trying to do but it takes time, and you may stumble a little along the way. Research proves that it takes most people four to five attempts to quit smoking, for example, but, if they keep trying, they eventually succeed. Develop a habit to never give up. This habit will do you much good in everything you pursue.

Chapter 7 Reference

Gumper, Bethany. 2005. "Pair Up for Better Results: Break Out of a Fitness Slump and Rediscover Your Motivation with an Exercise Partner." *Shape*. March. Health Publications. findarticles.com (accessed June 17, 2010).

8—Cycle Three

Chains of habit are too light to be felt until they are too heavy to be broken.   —WARREN BUFFET

Cycle Three Nutrition: Fat and Salt Reduction

To Do—

- *Reduce the amount of animal fats and butter you consume.*

- *Switch to healthier vegetable, olive, or nut oils.*

- *Reduce total salt intake.*

- *Avoid eating in restaurants.*

- *Maintain Cycles One and Two nutrition requirements.*

This is a six-week cycle broken up into two phases, each three weeks in duration, which will focus on developing a habit to prepare and consume lower fat meals and to reduce your sodium intake.

Unlike sugar and bread habits that can be very difficult to alter, your habit of consuming highly fattening foods can be softened and altered rather easily. Olive oil, canola oil, vegetable oils, and nut oils taste great, and you will find it fairly easy to use them in place of animal fats, butter, or lard. Butter Buds is a good artificial butter flavoring I use a lot. You also need to pay attention to the natural foods that contain saturated fats, such as chicken, beef, and pork. You are allowed to eat these foods, but try to make them as low fat as possible (see below).

Also, there are many alternatives to table salt currently available and while, at first, lowering your salt may be tough, your body craves health and will adjust very quickly.

Reducing Fat

During the first three-week part, please switch to 2% milk. The main thing to avoid during this phase will be any foods containing the words "partially hydrogenated vegetable oils," which is another name for trans-fatty acids. Many foods say "trans-fat free" but still contain partially hydrogenated fats. By law, the FDA allows any foods containing 0.5 grams or less to round down. However, according to the Harvard School of Public Health (2010), replacing 7 grams of carbs with just 4 grams of trans fat nearly doubles your risk for heart disease.

Many top nutritionists and medical authorities believe trans fats are one of the most harmful dietary substances you can consume. It is true that trans-fatty acids exist in nature and are found in very small quantities in deer, goat, sheep, beef cattle, and dairy cows; however, the manufactured version has a different chemical configuration than the natural trans fat.

Although the introduction of trans fats was a dream for the fast-food and the food-processing industries, more and more studies are showing that they are very bad for human consumption. Not only do they increase LDL (bad cholesterol) levels, they also decrease HDL (good cholesterol) levels. In 2002, the National Academy of Medicine stated that the only safe level of trans fat in the diet is zero (Center for Science in the Public Interest). In January 2006, new rules went into effect requiring companies to show trans fat content on nutrition labels (NIH). Again, the key words to watch out for and avoid are "partially hydrogenated oil" (of any kind) or "shortening."

The best way to avoid consumption of trans fat and the overconsumption of saturated fat is by preparing your own meals, but you can follow this new rule at delis or sandwich shops if you're careful. The body adapts to reducing unhealthy fats very quickly. Over time, Healthy Habit Plan followers develop increased sensitivities to greasy meals, complaining mostly of indigestion or sluggishness.

Remove skin and cut any visible fat off chicken, pork, and beef; when cooking ground meat, brown first, put in a colander, and then use hot water to rinse out the fat. (Also rinse out the pan if the recipe calls for you to continue with the same pan.) Choose reduced fat sandwich meats. Switch to liquid oils only for cooking, such as canola, olive, vegetable, and nut oils. Toward the end of this cycle, you will need to switch to 1% milk.

Throughout the entire cycle, avoid all kinds of margarines or shortening. These are basically solid blocks or tubs of trans fat. The rule of thumb: if it's solid when cold and liquid when hot, don't eat it. The only exception I make is natural butter. While butter is high in saturated fat, it is also natural and therefore recognized by the body. Just minimize your intake of butter. For example, you should avoid putting on more than ½ teaspoon per piece of toast and use Butter Buds instead of the real thing when cooking. It's a concept you can apply to all things on which you put butter. Remember, all you need is a taste, not a whole mouthful.

Sodium Reduction

In the second three-week phase, we will focus on lowering sodium (salt) content. Most Americans consume between 5,000 to 6,000 milligrams (mg) of sodium a day. The FDA generally recommends we keep our intake between 1,800 and 2,300 mg of sodium. This can be extremely difficult, and rather than trying to count milligrams, the easiest way to reduce sodium intake is to prepare all your meals at home and to avoid restaurants and processed foods. By now, you should be doing this anyway, but in this cycle, all restaurants and pre-made frozen meals are not allowed. The salt in homemade meals is miniscule when compared with restaurant food but still, for this cycle you will need to use a salt alternative such as AlsoSalt.

Too much sodium causes the body to retain fluid, which causes the heart to work harder and produces symptoms such as swelling and shortness of breath. For many, too much sodium could lead to high blood pressure, a risk factor in heart disease and stroke. It has also been linked to stomach cancer, kidney stones, osteoporosis, and worsening of asthma. Having said that, some salt is necessary for your body to function. Salt regulates blood pressure, aids in mineral transfer, and is the main component of the body's extracellular fluids; but the amount we need is minimal.

A Note on Sodium

A study conducted by Dietary Approaches to Stop Hypertension (DASH) found that cutting sodium to 1,500 mg lowers nearly everyone's blood pressure. The benefits of sodium restriction were especially striking when combined with a diet high in fruits, vegetables, whole grains, and low-fat dairy products. How striking, you ask? Individuals who consumed the least amount of sodium along with this type of diet dropped their systolic pressure (the top number) by an average of 11.5 millimeters of mercury (mm Hg).

Sodium can be found in many foods and in items with which we cook. Refer to the list below to educate yourself about where sodium could be sneaking into your diet.

Salt (sodium chloride)—table salt.

Monosodium glutamate (MSG)—common seasoning used in restaurants, hotels, at home, and in many packaged and processed foods.

Baking soda (sodium bicarbonate)—used in baking and cooking; sometimes used for indigestion. 1 teaspoon contains 1,000 mg of sodium.

Baking powder—leavening for quick breads and cakes; contains baking soda and acidic salts.

Other sodium compounds and where they can be found:

Disodium phosphate—processed cheeses and quick-cooking cereals.

Sodium alginate—chocolate milks and ice creams; used to create that smooth texture.

Sodium benzoate—relishes, sauces, and salad dressings; a preservative.

Sodium hydroxide—used in the processing of foods such as olives and certain fruits and vegetables (will not be found in fresh fruits and vegetables).

Sodium nitrate—cured meats and sausages; a hidden culprit for many migraine sufferers.

Sodium propionate—pasteurized cheese and some breads and cakes; used to inhibit mold growth.

Sodium sulfite—used in the processing of foods such as maraschino cherries and glazed or crystallized fruits before they are artificially colored. Can also be found in dried fruits as a preservative.

> **Habit Helper—**
>
> *Completely eliminating baking soda and baking powder would be nearly impossible, especially if you're an avid baker. I don't, and I do not expect you to. The goal here is not elimination, but rather reduction.*

I am not suggesting that you stop eating the above items. The purpose is to educate you on the foods that tend to contain high amounts of sodium. Read the label and select lower sodium versions of everything you buy. Be very wary of frozen dinners. These items can contain as much as 2,000 mg of sodium in one meal. If you're like many people and have a "salt tooth," use the Healthy Habit Plan approach, meaning, if you can't have it, find a healthy alternative to satisfy your cravings. I have listed some below.

Salt Alternatives: Having Salt without the Sodium

Since the hypertension epidemic, many salt alternatives have hit the market, and they are a great way to get the flavor and cooking benefits of salt without the worry of consuming too much sodium. Most alternatives use the compound potassium chloride. However, this compound, while handy, should be used in moderation and should not be used by anyone with heart or kidney disease. Read the label for a complete list of warnings. I recommend a salt substitute known as AlsoSalt. AlsoSalt uses a different, patented combination of potassium and L-lysine (an essential amino acid). The mixture of the two masks the bitterness. AlsoSalt can be used for cooking, baking, and sprinkling.

Cycle Three Nutrition—
Frequently Asked Questions

1. **How do I watch my fats when I eat in a restaurant?**

   Many restaurants use a lot of butter when cooking vegetables and meats, and most don't cut the fat off the meats either. Make sure to tell the waiter no butter or lard! Foods fried in animal fats are also not allowed. However, if the foods are fried in lower calorie liquid canola oil, vegetable oil, olive oil, or nut oil, then it is allowed, assuming all excess oil is drained or blotted off.

2. **If I use only a little bit of fat, is it okay?**

   It will be impossible to consume no fat at all, and it is unhealthy to not have any fat. I am mainly trying to alter your taste buds and your sensitivity to the overconsumption of saturated and trans fats. If you frequently eat meals high in these fats, it could possibly retard the habit-altering process. You are welcome to lighten up a bit on your saturated fat restriction once a week or so, but only after you have completed Cycle Three. After this, you will find that high-fat meals have a greasy, almost rancid taste and will often cause indigestion.

3. **May I still eat sugar-free candy bars and ice cream in this cycle?**

Unfortunately it's time to say good-bye to many of these little treats that I allowed you to consume while altering your sugar habits. These snacks, although low in carbohydrates and sugar are often extremely high in trans fat and saturated fats and indulging in them is definitely not healthy for long term. I use low-fat, sugar-free, high-fiber cereals with a little Stevia to satisfy my sweet tooth. Sugar-free hot chocolate is a low-fat, low-calorie snack that is excellent for dessert (watch out for the ones with trans fat). Whole fruit is, of course, the best choice for dessert. Craving sweets is 100% natural. Before there were such things as Twinkies and chocolate cakes, our sweet cravings insured that we ate plenty of fruit so, in a way, our sweet tooth aided in health. Fruit is the dessert Mother Nature intended us to consume. On your free meal after this cycle, partaking once a week in any kind of dessert should not do you much harm, but you may be surprised to find that you will probably be wishing you were eating an apple or strawberries instead of that chocolate bar.

4. **Why do you allow avocados, nuts, fish, olive oils, and peanut oils? They are often very high in fat.**

These foods are high in healthy fats and contain essential fatty acids that have been proven to be healthy for your heart. The goal is to reduce the saturated animal fats and trans fats. Just don't go overboard on cutting out all fats.

5. Do I need to use egg whites instead of whole eggs?

I don't require it. Eggs, although high in cholesterol, are low in saturated fats. The jury is still out on whether cholesterol-containing foods raise your cholesterol, and there is greater evidence that your cholesterol is affected by saturated fats and trans fat. The yolk in eggs contains more than 40% of the egg's protein and nutrients, but if you would prefer, you may use egg whites instead.

6. May I use a cholesterol-lowering margarine?

Popular cholesterol-reducing margarines contain natural substances derived from corn and beans called *sterol* and *stanol esters,* which have been proven to reduce blood cholesterol levels. They do this by interfering with the absorption of dietary cholesterol from the small intestines. The consumption of these supplements does not affect triglyceride or HDL levels. However, certain brands do contain a small amount of trans-fatty acids (see ingredients list), so take care to select ones that don't.

7. Do I really have to avoid all restaurants?

Yes, unless you personally know the chef and can guarantee he or she is not putting a tremendous amount of salt in the recipes or will reduce it just for you. Many restaurants use pre-made sauces and gravies, and frozen meats. These are extremely high in sodium. If you must eat out, pick a restaurant of higher scale if possible. It's easier to tell the waitress exactly what you want when you're paying a little more for your meal, and they're more likely to make accommodations for you. Typically, if you try to get picky and start demanding low-sodium meals at Joe's Grease Shack or The Feedlot

Saloon you'll just get a smirk and a "sure thing" but then end up with a salt bomb.

8. Why don't you totally eliminate salt like you do sugar?

Sugar would be healthy only in its natural state, which would mean actually chewing on the sugar stalk. When it comes to sodium, however, we all need it just to live, and it would be impossible and unhealthy to eliminate *all* sodium from your diet. The goal here is to develop a taste for the natural flavor of food without the added salt.

Cycle Three Recipes

PORK CHOPS WITH APPLES AND ONIONS

4 center cut pork chops, butterflied
2 large onions, sliced
3 apples, peeled, cored, and sliced
4 Tbsp canola oil, divided
2 Tbsp olive oil
3 Tbsp dry white wine
½ tsp crushed, dried rosemary
salt alternative and pepper to taste

Cut all visible fat from pork chops. Heat 2 Tbsp canola oil in nonstick skillet. Add pork chops. Cook on medium high until chops are browned on both sides and cooked through. In a separate skillet, heat the remaining canola oil. Add onions and sauté until onions are soft, about 4 minutes. Add apples. Add olive oil, salt alternative, and pepper to taste. Sauté onions and apples until onions are brown and apples are soft, stirring often. Add wine and rosemary. Cook for 1 to 2 minutes longer. To serve, spoon onion mixture on top of pork chop. (Peas are a great side item to this dish.) Be sure that total vegetables and meat are in equal proportions.

Makes 4 servings

FIRST PLACE CHILI

2 lbs lean ground beef
1 (16 oz) jar of Pace picante sauce
1 (12 oz) can Hunts diced tomatoes with celery, bell peppers, and onions
1 (12 oz) can pinto beans, drained and rinsed
1 pkg Williams chili seasoning (or any chili seasoning with no salt added)

Brown ground beef in 4-quart pot. Rinse away all fat by putting cooked meat in a colander and rinsing with very hot water. Be sure to rinse out the cooking pot as well. Return meat to pot. Add all remaining ingredients and simmer on low for at least 20 minutes, stirring occasionally. The longer the chili simmers, the more the flavors blend.

Makes 6 to 8 servings

OLIVE OIL BAKED POTATOES

2 medium-sized potatoes (russet, sweet, or red skin)
1 Tbsp olive oil
½ tsp salt alternative
½ tsp pepper

Preheat oven to 375 degrees. Split potatoes in half lengthwise. Place in gallon-size plastic bag or large mixing bowl. Add olive oil, salt substitute, and pepper. Toss to coat the potatoes with the seasonings. Place, cut side down, on a large baking sheet. Bake for 30 minutes or until potato is soft and cut side is browned. Serve as a side dish.

Makes 2 servings

Cycle Three Nutrition Habit Test

The Habit Test is something that makes this book unique. It is important that you do not move ahead in the cycles until you are certain that you have developed truly negative reactions to your once-favorite, but unhealthy, foods. Although you have been using motivation to help get you through this cycle, it is now time to allow your newly established habits to take over. People often have no idea how great an impact the foods they consume have on how they feel physically and mentally.

To take the test, you are to consume a large quantity of the food that you have been avoiding. A good test after Cycle Three would be to eat a large order of French fries or onion rings. The point here is to gauge your reaction—the stronger the reaction, the stronger the developed habit.

This test can and probably will be uncomfortable but I feel it is necessary to ensure that you will not be relying on willpower alone as you move forward. After you consume your forbidden food, I want you to wait thirty to forty-five minutes and then answer the questions below. It is critical that you answer honestly because your outcome will determine whether you are ready to move on to the next cycle.

1. *Did you enjoy the taste of your forbidden food?*
   A. Yes, I loved it and missed it. (1 point)
   B. No, it tasted horrible. (3 points)
   C. It was alright but not what I remember. (2 points)

2. *Did you have any mild stomach aches or cramps?*
   A. No, not at all. (1 point)
   B. Yes, I did experience a little stomach pain. (3 points)
   C. A little discomfort, but not much. (2 points)

3. *Did you have severe reactions such as diarrhea or vomiting?*
   A. I felt bad but did not get sick. (2 points)
   B. Yes, I threw up (or got diarrhea). (3 points)
   C. I experienced no severe side effects. (1 point)

4. *Did you really crave your forbidden food?*
   A. No, not at all. (3 points)
   B. Yes, I really looked forward to my forbidden food. (1 point)
   C. A little, but not as much as I used to. (2 points)

5. *Did you experience any lethargy?*
   A. Yes, a lot. (3 points)
   B. No, not at all. (1 point)

C. A little, but not much. (2 points)

6. **Did you experience unusual chest pressure after the consumption of your forbidden food?**
    A. Some, but not much. (2 points)
    B. Yes, a lot. (3 points)
    C. No, not at all. (1 point)

7. **Did you feel depressed after the consumption of your forbidden food?**
    A. Yes, I did feel depressed. (3 points)
    B. No, not at all. (1 point)
    C. I felt a little down, but not much. (2 points)

8. **Did you feel sudden restlessness or anxiety after the consumption of your forbidden food?**
    A. Yes, I did. (3 points)
    B. No, not at all. (1 point)
    C. I felt a little anxiety, but not much. (2 points)

9. **Did you feel cranky or moody after your forbidden food?**
    A. A bit, but not much. (2 points)
    B. Yes, very cranky. (3 points)
    C. No, I was in a great mood. (1 point)

10. **Did you even want to splurge today?**
    A. Yes, a lot. (1 point)
    B. No, not at all. (3 points)
    C. A little, but not much. (2 points)

Scoring Your Nutrition Test

If you scored 24 to 30, this is good news. It means you have developed a physical need to avoid the forbidden food. Not only have you developed a real sensitivity, but you have also lost your cravings and taste for it. To keep your sensitivity at high levels, please have only one free meal a week. You may not even crave it, but *do not overindulge* or you could experience very uncomfortable side effects.

If you scored 17 to 23, then you need to add another two weeks to your cycle. This is not a bad thing; it just means that your body is trying to hold on to some of its old habits. It is not unusual for people to need to extend the cycle for a couple of weeks. This score still means you have at least *started* to experience some negative reactions to fats and salts, so you're heading in the right direction.

If you scored 10 to 16, you need to find out if the forbidden food is sneaking into your diet somewhere, intentionally or not. When you get a score this low it means your body is having trouble building sensitivity. Don't get frustrated, you just need to take a look at your diet and really see if there is anything that could be disrupting the habit-altering process. What you need to do is add three weeks to Cycle Three and then take the test again. After that, you should at least score in the 17-to-23 range. Don't cheat! Consistency is the key.

Cycle Three Fitness

To Do—

- *Find more intense group training classes or increase the number of times you attend your current class.*

- *Hiring a personal trainer is optional at this time.*

- *Continue with your Cycle One activities on days you are not in class.*

> **Habit Helper—**
>
> *You should commit more to your chosen activity—sign up for tournaments, walks, and events of various sorts. Have a goal or something to work toward. This will take stress off your motivation.*

This cycle is almost the same as the Cycle Two exercise activities except for a few important things. Continue with motivating sport and hobbies that interest you, and consider increasing your obligation to these enjoyable activities. Enter some tournaments, or sign up for city walks and runs (in a group only) with friends. In this phase you can also up your commitment to weight training by stepping out of the group training atmosphere and hiring a one-on-one personal trainer. You can also move to high-intensity or advanced group training classes or Level 3 Activities. A minimum of one Level 3 and two Level 2 activities are required per week. You can do more, but don't do less; for example, don't take any days completely off. Plug in at least one Level 1 activity on days when you're not pursuing Level 2 and 3 workouts.

Level 3 Activities

- *Advanced or high-intensity group training classes*

- *Sport and hobbies, competitive-based activities*

- *Running in groups, rowing or cycling clubs*

- *Classical workouts, but only with a personal trainer*

Activities Not Allowed

- *Classical solo gym workouts* (will be allowed at Level 4)

- *Home workouts of any kind* (will be allowed at Level 4)

- *High-intensity solo cardio workouts such as solo running or cycling* (will be allowed at Level 4)

Cycle Three Fitness— *Frequently Asked Questions*

1. **Why can't I go running or cycling alone? I enjoy these activities!**

   This kind of solo, high-intensity cardio workout is not allowed in this cycle. It is not only the intensity of these activities that make them Level 4 but also the motivational factor. It takes a tremendous amount of discipline and willpower to stay consistent with these types of workouts, especially if you're new to fitness or are resuming activities after a lengthy time off. Many people say they enjoy these activities, and that's great, but often people underestimate how intense they can be, especially if they haven't done them for a long time.

   If you said you enjoy these activities, what does that

mean? Does that mean you are currently doing them now, or are you relating your great running experience back to when you ran track in high school? Have you ever been truly consistent, or are you off and on with your running, cycling, or other solo cardio program? Also, how intense are you? Is it a stroll or are you actually sweating and breathing hard? Answer these questions to yourself and be honest. If you're one of those who truly have been consistent with your solo workouts then that is awesome. That means you have already developed a "need" for exercise. For people like you, remember the Healthy Habit Plan is a philosophy, and it can be tailored to fit your needs. But for the rest, I suggest you follow the cycles to the letter.

2. What's the number one exercise you recommend in this cycle?

Group training, without a doubt! It's great for your body and doesn't take up a lot of motivational fuel. A favorite physical hobby or sport comes in at a close second.

3. What if Level 3 activities are too hard for me?

Slow down and stop them immediately. If you try to tough it out you could develop a negative mental connection, and you will start to associate exercise as painful, too challenging, and boring. This can be avoided by moving more slowly and allowing your mind and your body to learn to want more volume and intensity with your exercise. So, for right now, stick with Level 2. Depending on your personal needs, you may not need to advance past Level 2 activities, but I encourage you to challenge yourself before making that decision.

Cycle Three Exercise Habit Test

You will take this Exercise Habit Test on the same day as your Nutrition Habit Test. You are to be extremely inactive that day, and at the end of the day take the test below. Answer the questions truthfully about how you felt during your sedentary day.

Be honest, because your score will determine whether or not you are ready to move forward. The goal is to establish a physical need to be active every day because well-established habits can last a lifetime.

Sleep is equally important. Make sure you are getting seven to eight hours of sleep a night. If not, all the exercise and nutrition in the world will do little to make you feel better.

1. *Did you feel lethargic today?*

   A. Yes, I did. (3 points)

   B. No, not at all. (1 point)

   C. A little, but not much. (2 points)

2. *Did you feel anxious or nervous today?*

   A. No, not at all. (1 point)

   B. A little, but it didn't bother me. (2 points)

   C. Yes, I did. (3 points)

3. *How was your concentration level?*

   A. I was a little scatterbrained today, but not a whole lot. (2 points)

   B. My concentration level was horrible. (3 points)

   C. It was perfectly fine. (1 point)

4. *Did you feel guilty for being so inactive?*

   A. Yes, I felt very guilty. (3 points)

   B. No, not at all. (1 point)

C. A little. (2 points)

5. *Did you feel hungrier than usual?*
   A. No, not at all. (3 points)
   B. Yes, a lot. (1 point)
   C. A little bit. (2 points)

6. *Did you really want to get up and do something active?*
   A. Yes, I did. (3 points)
   B. I could have gone either way. (2 points)
   C. No, I enjoyed lying around all day. (1 point)

Scoring Your Exercise Test

If you scored 15 to 18, then congratulations; you are becoming habitually healthy. Your mind and body now need activity. Soon, you will become more and more "addicted" to physical activity with more intensity. More intensity means more muscle, more burned calories, and an athletic body.

If you scored 10 to 14, then you're heading in the right direction. Don't get frustrated! Everyone develops habits at a different pace. Many things, like past activity experience, genetics, diet, and more, play a part in your overall fitness level, as well as how quickly you adapt to physical change. Don't be in a hurry. Stay with this cycle for another two weeks and then take the test again.

If you scored 6 to 9, then something is interfering with the habit-altering process. Before you get frustrated, honestly answer these questions:

- *Are you following the activity guidelines exactly?*

If not, then you are probably burning yourself out. Remember, advanced workout routines require a real habit for exercise in order to be consistent. Anyone can work out hard for a week but you've got a bigger prize in mind—habits. *Slow way down!*

• *Are you consistent with your activity requirements?*

Just like the diet section, for a habit to be established, consistency is everything. Some people like the concept of the Healthy Habit Plan but are not motivated enough to wholeheartedly pursue it. Unfortunately, where there is no motivation, there is no real consistency. If you're having trouble being consistent, make sure you are moving slowly and doing activities you enjoy.

• *Are you eating properly?*

Make sure you are following the nutrition guidelines perfectly as you move through your cycles. If you are developing a habit for intense physical activity while leaving your eating habits untouched then this is counterproductive. The more active you are, the higher quality food and energy your body will need.

If you answered "no" to any of the above questions, add three weeks to your current cycle and then take the test again. This does not mean you have failed, it just means your habit of being sedentary is fairly ingrained. Don't fret. It takes time to change your habits.

The only way to beat a habit is with another habit. This is exactly what we are trying to do but it takes time, and you may stumble a little along the way. Research proves that it takes most people four to five attempts to quit smoking, for example, but, if they keep trying, they eventually succeed. Develop a habit to never give up. This habit will do you much good in everything you pursue.

Chapter 8 References

"Fats and Cholesterol: Out with the Bad, In with the Good." 2010. Harvard School of Public Health. www.hsph.harvard.edu/ (accessed June 17, 2010).

"NAS Panel: Only Safe Intake of Trans Fat is Zero." 2002. Center for Science in the Public Interest. July 10. www.cspinet.org (accessed June 17, 2010).

National Institutes of Health. 2006. "Your Guide to Lowering Your Blood Pressure." No. 06-4082. U.S. Dept of Health and Human Services. Originally printed 1998; revised April 2006.

9—Cycle Four

Excellence is an art won by training and habituation. We do not act rightly because we have virtue or excellence, but we, rather, have those because we have acted rightly. We are what we repeatedly do. Excellence, then, is not an act but a habit. —ARISTOTLE

Cycle Four Nutrition: Calorie Counting

To Do—

- *Learn to write down and monitor your calorie intake.*

- *Learn how to calculate the calories in your homemade meals.*

- *If additional weight loss is required, calculate your daily calorie requirements and reduce your total calorie intake.*

- *Maintain Cycles One, Two, and Three nutrition requirements.*

This cycle is unique from the others because of the simple, straight-forward requirement: counting calories. The more advanced you get in health, the simpler things get—and this cycle proves it.

For the next six weeks all I want you to do is count your daily calories. Every time you have a meal, every time you snack, every time you have a two-calorie mint or a piece of gum, you write it down. You've got to be attentive to detail but here's the deal, I am not asking you to reduce your calories, at least not yet. All I want you to do during this month and a half is to be aware of what you're eating and how much you're eating, and to learn how to count the calories.

Since, by this point, you should be eating high-quality food and have a habit for activity, your weight loss should continue regardless.

Calorie Counting: The Forbidden Words

Counting calories . . . *sigh*. I remember talking to a publisher years ago who specialized in health books. He told me those two words are fitness-book poison, and he was probably right. Over the last decade, there have been many diet books that have made it to the best-seller list not only because they probably followed this publisher's advice but because they took it a step further: ***Never count calories again!*** . . . ***Forget calories!*** . . . ***It's all about the carbs*** . . . or, ***It's all about the fat*** . . . or my favorite ridiculous claim, ***It's not what or how much you eat but when you eat!*** Simply put, counting calories seems to be one of the most-feared and horrible things a person has to do on a health program. I've met clients who have no problem giving up sugar, eating healthier, and even exercising strenuously, but getting them to even consider monitoring their caloric intake is like asking them to pull teeth with a pair of rusty pliers. Tell fitness newbies they need to start writing down everything they eat, and they oftentimes begin to sweat harder than the contestants on *The Biggest Loser*. Tell them they might need to buy food scales and weigh their food, and that's when they head for the hills.

Years ago at my gym, I found that about 85% of clients would balk when I asked them to start weighing their food. It's that intimidating for so many people. Why is this? The exact reason probably differs among people, but I imagine it's similar to being reluctant to getting on the scale. There's a fear of learning the truth or being held accountable. It never bothered me that much, but for others, it was often a deal breaker. Because of this, over the years I have formatted the Healthy Habit Plan cycles to allow a person to lose on average a couple of pounds a month without counting calories . . . at first. Simple math allows most people to easily see changes in their weight in the beginning cycles because we are addressing the big issues. Cycle One, on singling out and dealing with a sugar habit, is often where people see huge weight loss without counting calories. It's no surprise considering that just 12 ounces of soda has 160 calories.

Learning how to eat more balanced meals and to treat carbs as a portion rather than an entire meal is also a sneaky way to get people to lose weight. Developing a sensitive stomach to greasy, fattening food also works well to decrease overall daily caloric intake, as does developing a physical and mental need to be active daily; but eventually, resistance is futile. At some point you will need to develop an understanding of the proper amount of food that will allow you to maintain a healthy weight. Health nuts and lean people have developed a habit of being able to eyeball the perfect portions for their body. They know two helpings of one food are fine but two helpings of another food may not be. They also tend to know instinctively when they have had enough to eat. They know when to put the fork down because they've learned to recognize when they want to continue eating only out of boredom or just enjoyment of taste.

Fitness and diet writers have tried desperately to find a way around the "forbidden" words—counting calories—and whole programs have been developed around the eyeballing method, or portion comparison approach, in which a deck of cards is roughly the size of your protein portion and the size of a DVD is a helping of veggies, and other such approaches. You likely know the routine. Others have tried to adopt the "instinctual feeling" method. The theory here is that your body instinctively knows when it's full, and if you only listen you'll know when to stop eating. This approach does work *but only for the habitually healthy!* You don't know what you don't know. People who are heavy don't have an instinctual mechanism that tells them they're full, at least not anymore, which is at least one reason why they're, well, heavy, and the portion comparison, or eyeballing method, is an unrealistic approach because study after study has proved time and time again that people are terrible at guessing their caloric intake. There are many reasons for this, but two of them are the size of the meal and where you're getting that meal. Let's go over them:

1. *Meal Size*

    A study by Cornell University found that it was the size of the meal, not the size of the person, that determined how people underestimate calories. "We found that the more people had eaten, the less accurate they were," said Wansink, lead professor in the study. "It did not matter whether the person was skinny or huge, male or female—the bigger the meal, the less they thought they ate." Therefore, because overweight people tend to eat more large meals, they underestimate their food intake more frequently (Lang 2006). This is an excellent case for avoiding buffets. Putting yourself in a position where you are faced with an excessive amount of food is a recipe for disaster.

2. *Meal Source*

    Consider a basic lesson in psychology and this next one should come as no surprise. Studies show that people tend to order more calories when they are at "healthy" restaurants. We all relax a little when we're at the local healthy sandwich shop, but perhaps we shouldn't, because when people let their guard down, they order up 131% additional calories when the main dish is positioned as healthy (UCP 2007). A perfect example of this is Subway's lower-calorie, six-inch sub sandwiches. "Eat Fresh" has a nice healthy ring to it, and a six-inch chicken breast on wheat is advertised to have 320 calories.

> ### Habit Helper—
>
> *Like the idea of getting your money's worth at a buffet? Pack your lunch instead! It's a great way to make sure you have a healthy meal while saving money and preventing temptation!*

Not bad, but that is the sandwich alone with no cheese and no condiments. Add cheese, mayo, chips, and a soda and you've more than doubled those calories. But people tend to still feel good about their lunch choice and to approach dinner with that skewed number of 320 calories in their heads.

It's healthy, so how can you go wrong? Considering that many salads available rival (and sometimes beat) the calories in burgers, it's not as hard to go wrong as you think. Remember, healthy still has calories; going to a healthy restaurant does not make lunch a free-for-all. You still need to be aware of what you're eating. Visit a calorie-counting website and look up some of your favorite "healthy" foods. You may be pleasantly surprised but you may be horribly surprised. Knowledge is power. Applied knowledge is supreme power. Learn what you're eating, and don't let down your guard just because a restaurant has "fresh" or "healthy" in its logo.

At this point, you're probably getting a little nervous because you know where this is heading, and you're right. But before you angrily dig through the cabinets for that ancient weight scale you bought back in the eighties to accompany your signed copy of *Stop the Insanity,* or before you just say, "Screw it!" and throw the book in the trash, I'm here to tell you that when it comes to counting calories, you have nothing to fear but fear itself. I'm going to put some common misconceptions of calorie counting to rest.

Myth 1—It's so impractical and time consuming.

If the year were 1986 when a basic word processor cost around 500 dollars, and a slow-as-molasses personal computer took two hours to boot up, and floppy discs were actually floppy, then maybe I'd be inclined to agree. If the year were 1990 and 95% of fast-food restaurants were still very secretive about their calories, then maybe I'd understand. Fast-forward twenty-five years to an age in which computers link up to this magical global thing called the Internet, to when new laws require every major restaurant to provide the energy content of their food, and to when, within minutes, you can log onto literally hundreds of calorie management websites that have thousands of fast-food and other restaurant calorie information (many of which are free), calorie counting is just not that big of a deal anymore. Considering that the iPhone offers hundreds of apps that do this exact thing proves that the world of calorie management is at your fingertips. Most people don't need to even open up their laptop computer.

What about weighing your food or calculating a proper meal? Isn't that still a big, time-consuming pain in the rear? Well, yes and no. I won't lie. In the beginning, weighing your food and trying to calculate a perfect 500, 600, or 700 calorie meal accurately is a little tougher especially if you've never done it before, but it's simply a matter of remembering the recipe and saving it on a spreadsheet. In the recipe box I keep on my computer, I have stored dozens of calorie-calculated meals from 500 to 1000 calories and everything in between.

Don't have (or want) a computer? Many libraries, colleges, copy service centers, coffee shops, and other public places have computers you can use. Some charge a nominal fee, but you can likely find access for free if you begin asking around. Perhaps a friend who has a computer would be interested and willing to explore calorie counting with you? Perhaps you use a computer at work for your job and could ask for permission to use it for this calorie-counting purpose during a lunch hour or after work? And as a last resort, there are books listing calories for given foods in given quantities, some of which also help walk you through some sample meal plans. Spend time browsing the library and bookstore shelves for one that looks accessible and usable to you. One last thought, if you have friends who are on, or who have tried, one of the current weight-loss programs, they may have been provided with ingredient and calorie information for many of the fast-food establishments, and perhaps they would be willing to share such a list with you.

Habit Helper—

Grocery stores can be a problem. Not only are there so many temptations to buy the wrong things to take home with you, there are so many choices of things to eat and drink right in the store. Grocery carts even have cup holders now, so you can consume calories without even thinking about them as you make your way through the store! Especially during the early stages of altering habits, be creative about grocery shopping. For example, focus only on the items on your list, choose the checkout counter that is candy-free, take a supportive friend or family member along with you, or even ask someone else to shop for the items on your list.

For success with the Healthy Habit Plan, you need to re-evaluate how you feel about counting and monitoring your daily energy intake. I remember training one woman who argued with me for weeks about beginning her calorie counting, telling me it was impractical and time consuming, yet this same woman (who happened to be an accountant) was ridiculously obsessive when it came to managing her finances. She would often brag that her checking account was always perfectly balanced to the very last cent yet, for some reason, it completely escaped her that she could apply that same obsession to her health. She eventually did and it was the last piece of the diet puzzle for her. She lost more than a hundred pounds and has kept it off. Calorie counting isn't a new concept I invented, of course, but what my program did was change the way she looked at those forbidden but very effective diet words.

Because of modern technology, counting calories is no longer an impractical thing to do, and even though in the beginning it might seem time consuming, counting calories is the most effective way on earth to lose weight. The numbers never lie. If weight loss is your goal, saying that counting calories is time consuming is like a med student saying that college takes up too much time. Every person I know who has lost weight and maintained it, has learned in one way or another to manage daily caloric intake. The Healthy Habit Plan allows you to lose weight without breaking out the food measures for as long as possible, but eventually it'll be time to face this, and you'll be rewarded when you do.

Myth 2—Calories don't matter.

In this world of low-carbohydrate diets, blood type diets, vegan diets, and boot camp "puke-in-a-bucket" fitness routines, we're told that the weight gain epidemic is due to everything from meat to carbs to your special metabolic type, but very few bring up the fact that most people just eat too much food. There is so much BS floating around about the root cause of weight gain that it's easy to get confused and want to point the finger at things that have nothing to do with it.

The misconceptions are so prevalent, I'm sure you've already heard many of them and you may be using some yourself. (It's okay if you are, it'll be our little secret . . . I won't tell.) What I'm talking about is when people blame weight gain on things like conventionally grown foods, corporations poisoning the "food well," red meat, their thyroid, or some other nonexistent genetic disorder rendering them helpless in the fight to lose weight. This is just a sampling; as a personal trainer, I have heard them all. It's actually common for people to tell me they consume less than 1,000 calories a day and still can't get their weight below 280 pounds. Now, I've trained hundreds of people and every single one of them is someone I have truly enjoyed knowing, but no one's body is defying the laws of physics. (Albert Einstein proposed the concept of mass-energy equivalence, which is related to the Law of Conservation of Mass-Energy.) Briefly, mass cannot be maintained without having the energy to do so. Mass and energy cannot be created or destroyed, they can only change form. It is literally a physical impossibility for someone's body to be able to sustain a weight of 280 pounds on 900 calories a day.

Let's remember, a calorie is just a measurement of energy. When you eat food, your body converts what it needs into energy to perform your daily tasks and the rest is either excreted or stored. Storage especially happens when there is an excess of energy coming in, and since energy cannot be destroyed it converts into mass, and that mass ends up on your hips. If you maintain a level of caloric excess, it's the very thing causing your weight to creep up. The good news here is that it works the other way, too. If it takes more energy (calories) to maintain an overweight mass than you are consuming, your body will then convert the extra mass it has back into energy to sustain itself, thereby causing you to lose weight. See how awesome that is? The only scientifically proven way to lose weight is to create a caloric deficit. You can do this by being extremely active, you can do it by intensely monitoring your caloric intake, but the best way is to do both.

Myth 3—It's what you eat that is important, not how much, so calorie counting is obsolete.

There is some truth to this but only in a roundabout way. When you eat naturally, which means foods you can grow, hunt, or pick off a tree, the choices are typically extremely nutrient rich and are thereby very filling, causing you to eat fewer calories in the long run. Protein and fiber, two ingredients that are typically abundant in fruits, vegetables, and lean meats, have been called Mother Nature's calorie controls. Basically it's difficult to eat too much chicken breast, fish, veggies, and fruit because of the wholesomeness. You get more volume for fewer calories.

What's interesting, though, is that you can take something as healthy as fruit and juice it, strip it from its fiber, and turn it into naturally flavored sugar water, whereas a whole orange has only about 5% fructose. To equal the sugar content found in a glass of juice, you would have to eat an incredible number of pieces of whole fruit—more than most people would ever want, which I hope demonstrates further why we need to choose whole fruits and avoid fruit juices.

Heavily processed breads, sugars, and other similar products have been so refined it's as if they've already been digested, which means we absorb them quickly and our bodies have a hard time registering that they're full. This is why you can have a 525 calorie, king-size Snickers bar and feel hungry twenty minutes later. Try having a 500 calorie chicken breast or scrambled eggs instead. You'll feel stuffed.

Science tells us that "calories in, calories out" is the only way to lose weight, and that, yes, technically someone can get fat eating healthy food; however, in my years of experience growing up in the health industry and working with thousands of clients, I have never seen this happen. So, why would I still recommend calorie counting? Because calorie counting encourages you to eat healthy choices and educates you not only on what type of energy you're putting into your body but also how much. It also encourages you to eat a more balanced and natural diet. It's virtually impossible to go on a low-calorie diet, eat unhealthy foods, and last longer than a week.

Which would you rather have: several helpings of fish, chicken, and lean meat; two or three servings of fruit; two or three servings of vegetables; a serving of some whole grain OR one piece of cherry cheesecake? If you said cheesecake then it means you're not yet ready to watch your calories, which is why I introduce it later in my program. Bottom line, the healthier you eat, the more you eat; the more you eat, the fuller you feel; and it's the feeling of hunger that scares people out of dieting. Learning how to count your calories teaches you that, with the right choices, you don't have to feel famished.

Myth 4—You don't have to count calories if you just eat a smaller portion of what you usually eat.

This is another popular method that seems to attract people. Eat what you want, just stop before eating too much of it. On paper this works, scientifically it works, yet realistically it's one of the most ineffective methods. Take a person who has no physical sensitivities to large quantities of sugar and fat, a distorted idea of what a proper portion is, and a well-practiced habitual pattern of overeating, and you can see why this approach is problematic.

In a perfect world, eating just one cookie would be easy, or having that one piece of birthday cake every once in a while wouldn't affect your healthy habits one bit. Happily munching on some of Grandma's pie every now and then would be fine but, in the beginning, it's just too hard to stop before you've had too much.

It's apparent with today's obesity epidemic that people can't stop. They just keep eating and eating. The Healthy Habit Plan philosophy is clear and simple: single out one bad habit at a time, put all your effort into it, eliminate it, and replace it with a healthier habit. Do the habitually healthy ever splurge, ever have a piece of cake or ice cream? Sure they do, but there's a difference; when you've developed a habit for a healthy lifestyle, you can use moderation but not in the way you think. Your healthy habits will force a form of moderation. If I have a piece of cake and really enjoy it (which is rare), I know I can't have seconds—not because I'm worried that I'll get fat but because I fear the consequences. Stomach ache, nausea, or just an indescribable feeling of *blah* will always happen if I overindulge in sugary, fatty foods. So I stop before I get there. Trust me, with healthy habits, you make that mistake only once. If the habitually healthy fall off the wagon, more often than not, they're sprinting to get back on as quickly as possible.

Myth 5—You have to count calories forever.

Counting your calories until the end of time probably sounds pretty awful, but you won't have to do it so precisely forever. In addition to being the most foolproof, effective method for weight loss that ever existed, calorie counting re-trains your opinions about proper food portions. After years of watching my caloric intake, I can now estimate, off the top of my head, how many calories a banana with a scoop of ice cream has. I can tell you how many calories are in two pieces of Papa John's pizza and a Coke. Even at a buffet, I can build a balanced meal that's roughly around 600 to 700 calories, and I don't go back for seconds because I *know* I don't need to. I am fully aware of how calorie dense some foods are, which is one of the biggest reasons for our obesity epidemic. Knowledge is power.

A recent study published in the *American Journal of Preventive Medicine* found that the act of writing down and monitoring your daily food intake doubles your weight loss results (Kaiser Permanente 2008). Now why is this? This is simply the power of awareness. It's late and you're thinking about going for that dish of ice cream, but instead you pull out your food diary and realize how much you've already eaten. Surprised, you shake your head and suddenly reach a moment of enlightenment, realizing that you don't want the ice cream because you're hungry, you want it for other reasons. Maybe it's because you're bored or because you just have this oral fixation when you're watching TV. You're feeling a little guilty and a little humbled because that mean dietitian down the street who told you that you are eating when you're not hungry was right on the money. So, you go surf the web, read a book, and then go to bed. You do this for a few weeks and are actually surprised when you realize you've lost ten pounds. You weren't on some new TV-guru-approved diet or any supplements. You didn't even increase your activity. You simply became aware of what you were eating.

Calorie counting is kind of like putting yourself in a time machine and traveling back to the beginning, back when you were a kid starting to learn about foods like meats and vegetables. It is about re-educating yourself from the ground up on how to eat properly. It is impossible to accurately estimate calories for a few months and not begin to understand just how calorically dense many of the foods out there are. Suddenly it makes sense why you carry around an extra ten, twenty, thirty, or even a hundred pounds. Calorie counting kills that little person inside your head who wants to stand up and scream, "It's not my fault!!" It is simply the ultimate weapon against denial.

Despite the un-marketability of using these words, it is time to pull out the food measurer and food diary and, after several months, you'll realize why this is such an important part of becoming habitually healthy.

So, here we go.

Counting calories isn't the easiest thing to do in the beginning. You can't expect it to be convenient or fun, at least at first. It's a hard skill to develop but you *can* develop it and like anything, if you do it long enough, it will become another little habit you do, like balancing your checkbook, and it will eventually teach you how to develop a low-calorie diet for yourself. The Healthy Habit Plan has a few secret weapons that have made the traditionally difficult, low-calorie diet easier to swallow.

Secret Weapon 1—Habit for eating healthier

This is the last cycle for a reason. By now I am hopeful you have developed an aversion to high-fat, high-sugar meals and developed an affinity for healthier options. This isn't just great, it's outstanding. However, the basic laws of thermodynamics are still in place. Technically, if you still have more weight to lose, it doesn't necessarily mean you're cheating. By now you shouldn't be able to cheat, but you could possibly be eating too many calories even if they are healthy. It is harder to do with healthy food but not impossible. Healthy carbs, fiber, and lean protein have a bigger nutrient bang for your calorie buck and help significantly with satiety, which means that your habit for eating right will be your secret weapon while counting calories.

Secret Weapon 2—Exercise and Activity

Exercise has a profound impact on the utilization of stored energies. Although exercise alone is not particularly effective for weight loss, research shows that combined with a low-calorie diet it increases the effectiveness dramatically. "In the midst of America's obesity epidemic, physicians frequently advise their patients to reduce the number of calories they are consuming on a daily basis. This research shows that simply dieting will not likely cause substantial weight loss. Instead, diet and exercise must be combined to achieve this goal," explained Judy Cameron, Ph.D., a senior scientist at Oregon Health & Science University's (OHSU) Oregon National Primate Research Center, a professor of behavioral neuroscience and obstetrics and gynecology in the OHSU School of Medicine, as well as a professor of psychiatry at the University of Pittsburgh. The regulation of free fatty acids, increased blood flow, better utilization of blood sugar, and increased glycogen storage capabilities are all things that exercise does that will aid you during a low-calorie diet. And remember, even though an increase in activity can lead to a higher appetite, *high*-intensity activity will *decrease* appetite.

More Tools to Help You Reach Your Goals

I know you're now ready to begin practicing the oldest, most effective way to lose weight that exists on the planet: calorie counting. But you need more tools because, like all the other cycles, before calorie counting becomes a habit, it will feel more like a chore. Grind it out and you will be rewarded. Just like riding a bike, it's a skill that will have you stumbling for a while, but when it clicks, it's easy and you'll be surprised by how effortlessly you can include it in your lifestyle. Here are some more tips to make calorie counting even easier.

Tip 1—Don't eat in restaurants very often

This is not an unbreakable rule, but if a restaurant does not provide calorie information, don't go. Also, even in the ones that do provide it, pay close attention to exactly what they're counting. They may leave off side items or condiments to get that number nice and low but then serve them to you when you order.

Furthermore, the calories they are advertising may be wrong. In a study conducted by Tufts University, researchers analyzed the calorie content of eighteen side dishes and entrees from several national sit-down chain restaurants, eleven side dishes and entrees from national fast-food restaurants, and ten popular frozen meals from supermarkets. Afterward, they compared their results with the calorie info listed on menus and labels. The study found that most of the information provided to the public was grossly inaccurate. For instance, the calorie claims made by the restaurants were found to be 18% less than the researcher's calorie content analysis. Additionally, two side dishes exceeded the restaurant's reported calorie information by nearly 200% while the calorie information reported by the packaged food companies averaged 8% less than the researchers' analysis (Tufts University 2010).

In franchises and corporations, the original recipes are created in their headquarters or research kitchen, and then passed down to all the franchisees or corporate restaurants where chefs in each individual restaurant are expected to recreate the dish exactly. The same way that rumors change when they are passed from ear to ear, so do recipes. One chef uses slightly more cheese and sauce, another chef adds more chicken and, in the hustle and bustle of a professional kitchen, the recipes get altered and calories shift.

The moral of the story is to avoid situations where you can't be sure about what you're eating. Dining in restaurants makes calorie counting extremely hard and, in some cases, impossible.

Tip 2—Get the hardware

- *Get a food scale, you will need it.*

- *Sign up for an online calorie-counting website (many are free) and get a calorie-counting book. I like* The Ultimate Calorie, Carb & Fat Gram Counter *by Lea Ann Holzmeister, RD, CDE. Heck, get two or three copies and have one at work, home, and in the car.*

- *Buy two blank diary books. One will be your food diary, an accurate, complete, blow-by-blow description of your eating life. The other will be your recipe book. Every time you make a perfectly balanced meal, you will write the recipe down, logging the calories per serving so you never have to calculate that meal again.*

- *Last but not least, purchase a body-weight scale and become friends with it every single morning.*

Tip 3—Learn the math

Don't worry if you flunked high school Algebra, counting calories is not that complicated. With a little attention to detail, you will be instinctively estimating calories in your head every time you grocery shop.

> **Habit Helper—**
>
> *While you're calculating calories, don't forget to take any oils or butters that you cooked with into consideration.*

First, it is important to establish some kind of serving size or size reference when you're doing your calculations. On prepackaged items, pay close attention to the serving size listed and measure that amount. If you are consuming more, you will need to multiply the calories accordingly. Likewise, if you are eating less, then the calories listed should be divided.

On some products, the list has very straightforward numbers such as "6 crackers per serving," in which case counting is a no-brainer. But on other products, all you have to work with is a number such as "120 calories per serving" and then another number that reads "approx. 6 servings per package." So it doesn't just come out and tell you how much to get. There are two ways to calculate here: you can either pour out the entire box and divide it into six equal servings, or you can use the weight measurement they have (usually milligrams or ounces) and weigh it on a food scale. Just to help you out, there are 30 milligrams per one ounce.

Never assume that just because something comes in a nicely sized, individual package that it is just one serving. Bottled juice is a perfect example. Very often, there are 2½ servings per bottle making that 150 calories shown on the label more like 375 calories. The dried noodles with the flavor packet that are so popular among college kids are another example. It's easy to assume there is just one serving per package but, in fact, there are two.

Tip 4—Basic food preparation

You will need some skills in the kitchen as well, and I will provide a few detailed, easy-to-make recipes as examples.

So, how do you calculate the calories in your homemade meals? It's not as hard as you think. The secret is to put the effort into it once and then write it down. That way, you'll never have to do it again, and preparing that particular meal gets easier every time. I have many of my meals on a spreadsheet on my computer so I can print them off and access them wherever I am.

Some meals are easier than others. For example, a meal consisting of a grilled chicken breast, a serving of peas, and a serving of baked sweet potatoes is relatively easy to measure, weigh, and calculate. But what about one-pot meals such as chili or your special, home-made spaghetti sauce? Here's how you do it: Add up everything—and I mean everything—that goes into the entire pot of food. Then (this is the only tough part), you will measure out how many cups, or eight-ounce measures, you have in the whole pot. You do this by getting a second pot or bowl and using a one-cup measure to scoop and count how many cups are in your dish. After that it's simple math. Here is an example using spaghetti sauce.

Spaghetti Sauce

1½ lbs lean ground beef	1160
1 Tbsp olive oil	120
1 cup onion, chopped	61
4 oz button mushrooms	40
58 oz Hunt's tomato sauce	195
1 cup Hunt's tomato paste	220
spices	0

Brown meat in large sauce pan. Drain and rinse meat with hot water, return to pan. Add olive oil, onions, and mushrooms. Cook until onions are translucent. Add tomato sauce, tomato paste, and desired spices. (I usually add about 1½ Tbsp of basil, 1 Tbsp oregano, ½ teaspoon each of rosemary, salt, pepper, and a dash of thyme. Also, about 1 Tbsp of minced garlic, which adds a negligible amount of calories). Simmer and serve over cooked pasta.

Makes 10 cups   1796 calories (180 calories per cup)

One cup of cooked spaghetti noodles is 198 calories, thus one cup each of pasta and sauce is 378 calories.

How to Lose Weight

As if this whole book wasn't about that very thing! There is a formula for calculating your caloric needs. It takes into consideration things such as your age, height, gender, and activity level. The easiest way to calculate your caloric needs is by finding a formula online. It's as simple as typing "calorie calculator" into your search engine. I personally like the one at www.dietblog.com. It lets you know how many calories you need to eat to maintain and how many you would need to eat to lose weight. This calculator uses the Mifflin formula, which currently appears to be one of the most accurate, predictive equations for both normal weight and obese individuals. Now, if you want to *lose* weight, put in the weight you *want* to be. For example: Watch every single thing that goes in your mouth and make sure your daily calories do not exceed this number. Do this and weight loss **will** happen.

Habit Helper—

Having trouble with mindless eating? Try this: Rubber mouth guards are available at almost every drugstore. Follow the instructions to shape it to your mouth and then wear it everywhere you go. Since you can't eat with it in, eating and snacking becomes a bit of an ordeal since you have to take out the mouth guard, eat, then rinse it off, and put it back in. This is a sneaky way to make sure you notice everything you eat. It can also work as a deterrent to keep you from snacking on unnecessary calories in the first place!

Cycle Four Recipes

Here are some more pre-calculated recipes to give you a head start. The calories are listed beside each item so feel free to adjust them up or down for your calorie requirements.

Fajitas (dinner size)

2 Mission brand low-carb, fajita-size tortillas   160

8 oz flank steak	426
4 tsp canola oil	106
½ cup Pace picante sauce	40
1 cup onions, sautéed	92
1 cup bell peppers, sautéed	38
½ cup reduced fat Sargento cheese	160
Dessert—1 cup fresh cantaloupe, cubed	56

Sauté flank steak in 2 teaspoons canola oil with desired spices. Sauté onions and peppers in separate pans in 2 teaspoons canola oil. Add ¼ teaspoon salt and pepper to each. Warm tortillas and roll steak, sauce, onions, peppers, and cheese inside.

Makes 2 servings   539 calories, each

Taco Salad (dinner size)

8 oz extra lean ground beef	386
2 tsp canola oil	53
1 cup fresh spinach	7
½ cup tomatoes, diced	19
½ cup onions, diced	30
½ cup Pace salsa	40
½ cup low-fat shredded cheese	160
2 oz baked Tostitos	220

Brown beef in 2 teaspoons canola oil and add desired spices. Place Tostitos in a bowl and add spinach on top of them. Spread meat, tomatoes, onions, salsa, and cheese over the spinach.

Makes 2 servings   458 calories, each

Chili for a Big Crowd

4 lbs extra lean ground beef	2072
2 cans pinto beans, rinsed	700
2 cans diced tomatoes with chiles	315
2 jars Pace salsa	420
1 pkg Williams chili seasoning	0

Brown beef in large pan. Add remaining ingredients. Simmer for at least 30 minutes, stirring occasionally. May be served with pasta, and/or other foods, to make a 3-way chili (protein, carbohydrates, and vegetables).

Makes 17 cups   206 calories per cup

Cheeseburger

6 oz lean beef patty	290
1 small whole wheat bun	120
2 slices fat free cheese	60
¼ cup spinach	1
1 slice onion	8
1 Tbsp pickles	4
2 slices tomato	7
1 tsp mayo	30
1 tsp mustard	4

Makes 1 serving   524 calories

Season beef and grill or broil until done, then assemble. I use spinach instead of lettuce because it is delicious and contains more iron, calcium, and antioxidants.

Banana Nut Muffins

3 very ripe bananas	315
6 oz plain, unsweetened yogurt	80
¼ cup buttermilk	24
2 Tbsp butter, melted	204
2 eggs	156
2 cups whole wheat flour	800
¾ cup sugar substitute	0
½ tsp salt	0
¾ tsp baking soda	0
1 oz chopped pecans	187

Preheat oven to 350 degrees. In a large bowl, mash bananas and stir together with yogurt, buttermilk, melted butter, and eggs. In a separate bowl, combine remaining ingredients. Add dry ingredients to wet ingredients and stir until just combined. Do not over-mix. Drop by spoonfuls into lined muffin pan. Bake for 20 to 25 minutes or until lightly browned and toothpick inserted in middle muffin comes out clean. Cool 10 minutes before serving.

Makes 12 muffins   147 calories each

Without nuts   131 calories each

Optional: sprinkle ½ teaspoon Butter Buds on top. This adds 17 calories to each muffin.

Cycle Four Fitness

To Do—

- *You are now free to pursue any kind of activity you want to,*
  as long as you are active every day.

This is the cycle in which Level 4 activities, such as home workout programs or working out alone in a gym, are allowed. You should already be at the point where you feel like you must do something active every day and, if you truly feel this way, then it means you're ready for this cycle. Understand that working out alone and having to push yourself takes a lot of effort and only the habitually healthy can do these workouts with proper intensity and consistency to see any results. Despite what I have said about most gym workouts, weight training and other classical gym workouts can build an incredible level of fitness. But don't count out other physical activities as well. I have met mountain climbers, surfers, martial artists, and avid hikers who have never stepped foot in a gym, and they too were fit and muscular.

Remember, attempt Level 4 activities only if you already have an established habit for exercise. Level 4 activities are not only physically tough but mentally tough as well and would be the kiss of death, in terms of building or maintaining a consistent workout, for anyone without established habits.

There are hundreds of different weight-training programs out there and most work, if you *do* them. This should not be a problem for the habitually healthy individual. Nothing physical is off limits anymore because you now work out not only because you want to but also because you have to. Get out there and find out what makes you fit, happy, and healthy. The world of fitness goes much farther than the typical health club scene. Good luck!

Habit Helper—

Circuit training (basically cardio with weights) is sometimes used by people trying to build muscle and lose weight. Unfortunately, you can't do both at the same time. Weight training builds muscle because the weights are heavy and the rest times are long. In circuit training, the weight is too light to get this strength benefit but it is great for cardio endurance. Both types of training are effective, but they should be done separately. Do a strength cycle with heavy weights for six weeks then follow it with a fat loss cycle using cardio. This will give you the best of both worlds.

Cycle Four Fitness—
Frequently Asked Questions

1. **That's it? No detailed fitness program?**

   No! I have left it more open on purpose. The Healthy Habit Plan is a health philosophy, something that will help you to mentally and physically develop the proper habits so that you can live a healthy lifestyle despite the temptations brought on by our often not-so-healthy environments. Many Healthy Habit Plan followers consider my book to be a health and fitness prequel, the missing first chapters of every other program. It is easy to show someone how to eat right or to exercise, in fact many already know how. Why people are not doing it, however, is the bigger concern.

2. Do I *have* to do Level 4 exercises?

Not if you consistently participate in at least Level 3 activities. There are also many Level 3 activities for which overall intensity can be increased, making it a Level 4—for instance, martial arts. These are considered multi-level activities. Other than that, your intensity level should be dictated by your goals and how you feel. When you develop a real need for exercise, which I'm hopeful you have by now, not only will you want to consistently exercise but you may find that your body will crave more intense activities. The Healthy Habit Plan is about being fueled by habits or the absolute need to eat healthy foods and to exercise. Don't force anything. If you don't feel like you need to work out harder, then don't. Level 3 activities are a great level for lifelong health.

Chapter 9 References

Kaiser Permanente. 2008. "Keeping A Food Diary Doubles Diet Weight Loss, Study Suggests." *Science Daily.* July 8. www.sciencedaily.com (accessed June 8, 2010).

Lang, Susan. 2006. "It's the Size of the Meal, Not the Size of the Person, that Determines How People Underestimate Calories, Cornell Study Finds." Chronicle Online. Cornell University. November 1. www.news.cornell.edu (accessed 2010).

Tufts University News Releases. 2010. "Study Examines Calorie Information from Restaurants, Packaged Foods." January 6. news.tufts.edu (accessed June 14, 2010).

[UCP] University of Chicago Press Journals. 2007. "You're Likely To Order More Calories at a 'Healthy' Restaurant." *Science Daily.* September 5. www.sciencedaily.com (accessed June 7, 2010).

10—*Wrapping Up*

Habit with its iron sinews, clasps us and leads us day
by day.   —ALPHONSE DE LAMARTINE

A Healthy Balance

Now that you've gone through the program, I am sending you out into
the world. My research suggests that when your meals are properly
balanced (protein and carbohydrates in generally equal quantities),
most people feel fuller and better overall. This is the Healthy Habit
Plan's recommendation but you should experiment as you move forward in your new, healthier lifestyle. If you do a lot of running, for
example, try a diet for runners. If you're an avid weight lifter, research
the many body-building nutrition programs available. You see, if you
look closely at the content of every sound, well-balanced diet out
there, most preach the same thing: whole grain, lean sources of protein, vegetables, whole fruits, and nuts. This author might lean more
toward a higher percentage of protein or more toward a higher percentage of carbs but, bottom line, the diets are all very similar. You'll

also notice that no diet recommends saturated fats, high sugar con-sumption, or refined foods. Pick any structured diet if you think this will help you with continual improvements. I strongly believe that if you eliminate the high-fat, high-sugar foods in your diet and eat plenty of protein, fruits, and vegetables, it's hard to go wrong.

The Reason for Health

He who has health, has hope; and he who has hope, has everything.   —ARABIAN PROVERB

At its core, the Healthy Habit Plan is similar to other sensible fitness programs that are available. It uses the same tools of calorie restric-tion, exercise, and instilling healthy eating in order to reap the physical benefits of being fit. The difference lies in the application. The process of slow habit alteration in combination with realistic motivation-spar-ing techniques gives this program a very high success rate.

But, getting healthy still takes work. This, and any other fitness program, will take a certain amount of commitment and with all the stresses of life, work, and family, I have often been asked, "Why, Wes? Is it really worth it all?"

Oftentimes when we grow older, get married or form committed relationships, and have kids and/or take on increasing responsibil-ity as adults, the desire to have those bulging biceps, flat abs, or shapely rear end no longer holds the importance that it once did, and perhaps this is justifiable. But if you look at it this way, you are looking at the gift of health at the surface level only, and it goes much farther than skin deep.

As a fitness professional who trains real people—hard-working regular folks who often work forty-plus hours per week, run businesses, and chase down children all day—I will tell you that the transformations I've seen are so much bigger and better than rippled abs and sculpted shoulders. It's the little things. It's the client who, despite his once-bad heart, can now play a little basketball with his kid in the driveway, it's the grandmother whose back and arms are now strong enough for her to pick up her grandkids, and it's the teenager who now has the confidence to go to that swim party and not worry about standing out as some Greek god, but to, instead, fit in and feel normal.

The gift of health goes so much farther than the "get buff" mentality and allows people to do the things they want to do. Health, to me, is seeing my sixty-year-old father still be fit enough to walk for miles and then climb a deer stand and hunt because that's his passion; it's seeing my grandma fit enough to spend hours in the garden, and it's watching my best friend being flexible and mobile enough to scoot and crawl and squat all over the place while fixing up his sports cars, because that's what he loves to do. It's being able to compete at and enjoy my martial arts year after year without major injury.

Physical fitness allows each of us to live our own unique flavors of life to our personal max, no matter what it is. So, to answer your question, "Why, Wes?" well, . . . I'll tell you why. Because I feel that our time on earth is sacred and precious, and if someone told me there was something I could do to give me more *quality* time on this earth to do the things I love and to be with the people I love, then I would be all for it. And if that thing is as simple as taking care of myself, like exercising and eating right then, yes, I say it's worth it; and I'll go so far as to tell you that I think you should take are of yourself, too.

A Final Tip

I want to thank you again for allowing me to guide you through the intimidating and often confusing world of health and fitness. It's a responsibility that I do not take lightly and because of this, I want you to know that the words on these pages, each and every one of them, have been a true labor of love for me.

My first coach told me so many years ago, "Wes, your clients can smell a rat. They know if you would rather be doing something else." I wrote down those words and hung them up in the office of my first gym. The weight room was a small, 250-square-foot room, and all I had was a lot of used free weights from my wife's boss who got them super cheap from another gym that was closing.

Fast-forward several years, sitting in my new gym I sometimes feel like I'm a million miles away from that old place, but I haven't forgotten it or those words that still hang on my wall. I always promised myself that the moment I started to lose passion I'd quit and become some- thing else, like maybe a Navy Seal or a cage fighter or a barber. Not because I'd want to but because I'd have to. Trainers and health gurus with no fire left in them are like pencils with no lead: it's just not going to work. Sure, they might have made it big and scored a profitable Yoplait yogurt or a supplement sponsorship, with a new line of frozen dinners to their name and their pretty face on the microwavable box, but in the end, that doesn't fool anyone. My sincerity is real because this is what I love, and I can't think of anything else I'd rather do than show people how they can unlock that inner health nut.

As a final point, I want to share something with you. I can't entirely take credit for coming up with the idea of habitual health. Benjamin Franklin, one of the most successful human beings who ever lived, took a similar approach more than 100 years ago. He called it his Twelve Virtues. He had a theory that if he singled out one bad habit at a time, he could conquer it and then move on to another one. Things like gluttony, alcohol, even sex were covered. Giving a week to each bad habit, he would go through them all, put his effort into turning each habit into a better one, and then start all over again. After showing this approach to a friend of his, that friend suggested he add another one, humility, of which his friend claimed Franklin had none. Franklin thought about it for a while but in the end went ahead and added a thirteenth virtue.

According to some of his writings, this approach worked very well for him as he was able to get better control of his health and his vices, all except for one. It was the last one, the thirteenth virtue. He said it was the only one he failed to change because he had decided he was simply not a humble person. But did he really fail? The only virtue at which he did not succeed was the thirteenth virtue; his friend's desire for humility was not his own. This brings me to my point. Franklin did not add the thirteenth virtue himself because he did not value that virtue, his *friend* did. In other words, Franklin did not want it in the first place and therefore did not put the effort into it.

If you do not *want* to change, if you don't feel you *need* to change, then there's nothing I, the Healthy Habit Plan, or anyone can do for you. Concerned friends and family can help push you to change, but the initial desire, the motivating desire, has to be there from within yourself.

My question to you is this: On your personal list of self-improvements, where does your health rank? Is it something you really want to improve or, much like Benjamin Franklin, is it your thirteenth virtue? Do *you* want it or do those around you want it for you?

When I first started practicing martial arts, there was such an air of mystery about them. The longer I practiced, however, the more the mystery and intimidation faded. I discovered that the reason martial artists were able to do such amazing things was because they pursued their sport each and every day. After doing it myself for a while, excellence and hard work wasn't something that I had to dig deep and strive for anymore; it was a habit, something that had become so ingrained in me that giving less than 100% effort would be harder. That's when I discovered there was more to the art than just discipline. Health and fitness is no different. Once the curtains are pulled back, it's just a bunch of work, both mentally and physically. I believe that if you follow a proper approach, hard work becomes second nature and positive results are inevitable.

Humans are creatures of habits. We instinctively seek out the familiar and whether that familiarity is running two miles a day, or smoking two packs a day, the psychology is the same. You have a choice. Right now, you have the power to change your habits, to become a healthier person, and this is better than any magic pill because unlike that pill, habitual health is real, and it is a part of each and every one of us. I wish you all healthy habits for life.

> Watch your thoughts; they become words. Watch
> your words; they become actions. Watch your actions;
> they become habits. Watch your habits; they become
> character. Watch your character; it becomes your
> destiny.   —FRANK OUTLAW

Appendix I—

Finding the Right Health Club
or Support Group

If you've skipped some of the earlier chapters let me reiterate a core Healthy Habit Plan philosophy: working out at home typically doesn't work. Finding another place to train at which you feel comfortable is very important. I want to assure you that despite anyone's past "bad gym" experiences, if you follow some of these tips, you'll have an easier time adhering to the exercise guidelines and will have a better experience.

Find a Place That Offers Group Training

From the giant mega gym to the little Jazzercise class that's been in that strip mall since the eighties, just about every kind of commercial gym offers some form of group training. Don't be glamorized by a gym with a lot of free weights and weight machines. For a beginner who has very little knowledge and experience in exercise technique and a limited amount of motivation, walking into a big gym and trying to follow the generic exercise workout on the clip board that the salesman gave you can be a frustrating experience. Not only do you not know how to work out, but even if you had the technique down, it's been my experience that a fitness newbie has a hard time pushing him- or herself at the proper intensity.

Group training, on the other hand, is extremely gentle on your motivation because all you need is enough gumption to get yourself there, and then follow the instructor. You might be ready to stop at rep ten on squats in a conditioning class, but when an instructor is yelling out *"Twenty"* and everyone else is at least trying, you'll push yourself harder than you ever would have at home or on your own on some leg extension machine.

The variety is great as well. You can choose from yoga, Pilates, group weight training, kickboxing, boot camp style, spin, Zumba, dance, aerobics, Jazzercise, and the list goes on nearly forever.

Find a Personal Trainer

Working out with a trainer is like group training on performance enhancements. A good trainer not only shows you proper form but also, more than anything, pushes you beyond what you could ever push yourself to do alone. There is a reason why even the fittest, strongest athletes in the world have their own trainers—they know even they could never work themselves as hard as a trainer can.

However, personal training can be expensive. Good trainers will price their services anywhere from $40 to $80 an hour (or more) depending on experience, education level, and where you live. An increasing number of personal training companies are countering this with a new way to train called "semi-personal," which means you share your session with up to three or so other people. That way, the cost is allayed a little, but the group is still a small enough for each participant to get a lot of personal attention. This is definitely something to think about.

Find a Specialty Gym

Do you find yourself just loving all the kickboxing classes? Many martial arts schools provide a variety of different kinds of martial arts fitness classes especially designed for those who want to experience the physical benefits of training without the contact. Classes range from cardio kickboxing to Tae-Bo-style classes.

If you're highlighting all the yoga classes at your gym, you won't have any trouble finding some private studios that do nothing but yoga.

Love those group weight-training classes but want to kick it up a notch and get a little stronger and receive more individual attention? Then smaller personal training studios with knowledgeable trainers offer a variety of private and semi-private sessions to meet any budget.

Dancing studios can turn your once- or twice-a-week fitness class into a serious, competitive hobby.

Years ago I had a client who had a passion for heavy lifting. I hooked him up with a power lifter friend of mine, and he began working out with these beastly looking guys in some warehouse downtown doing hardcore stuff like sled dragging, sprints, dead-lifts, and bar bending bench presses. He now competes in power lifting.

Some trainers shrug off group training classes as "stupid and ineffective"—don't listen to them. Group training can be a gateway to so much more.

Laugh Off the Criticism

This might not be much of a problem if you're a woman, but if you're a guy, there seems to be a negative stereotype about taking a group training class. People seem to think there's something strange about taking a spin class or a boot camp class with a bunch of ladies.

(Personally, I've always thought that being surrounded by women wearing spandex was a good thing.) It's true that almost all styles of group training are dominated by women, but you would be crazy to think this decreases the effectiveness of it. Next time one of your macho "home workout" or "weight training only" buddies teases you about going to group training, take a real good look at your friend's physique and the consistency of his routine. If he has to brush off three inches of dust every time he hits the free weights in his garage, or rubs his massive beer belly as he laughs at you going to spin class, use common sense. Who's the one looking silly?

Go Outside

Hate the gym scene? You can still work in a group outside. Most towns have running clubs, cycling clubs, and even rowing clubs. As long as you still work out in a group, you never have to step foot in a gym. I've found that those in running clubs have this bond that I suppose can be forged only by the experience of running or cycling miles and miles together in windy, cold, or hot weather. You miss more than a day, these people will be calling you and telling you to get your butt back in gear. It's a great support group. My gym ran a running club for years with lots of success.

Try Old-Fashioned Aerobic Studios

It may feel like stepping back into an eighties time capsule when you go into a Jazzercise class a few times a week, but you'll see results and you might actually enjoy it. Don't underestimate a good old-fashioned aerobics class. The instructors and the pace range from slower, low level to super high intensity. Don't let all the modern health gurus tell you that aerobics is out and weight training is in. Just like one of my mentors told me years ago, "You can go outside and chase your beagle in your backyard for forty-five minutes and get a great workout. The secret is in packaging the exercise so the client can take it down." What my coach was trying to explain to me was, when it comes to burning calories, movement is movement. Find some type of movement that you like.

Look Online for Support

In the twenty-first century, weight-loss support is available all over the Internet. Remember, when it comes to altering your habits, you simply can't have too much support and positive energy around you. You must drown yourself in it. It's a great feeling to come home after a hard workout and see in your in-box several e-mails from other people going through the same thing you are.

Appendix II—

For Friends and Family:

How to Support a Loved One on the Journey to Health

I'm serious. Have all your friends and family members, the ones who are around you the most, read this. It's not for you.

It's hard to believe but many people are so afraid of change they don't even like seeing it in others. This is something very few people like to talk about in fitness and diet books, but it's the truth. Oftentimes the people we love the most can be the most effective at sabotaging our attempts at life changes. I've seen this so many times I've lost count.

It's been my experience that most loved ones are not doing this out of spite or meanness; it's more of a subconscious thing. Maybe you're upset because they're not enjoying the same things with you anymore, or perhaps their initiative to change their life has made you feel guilty that you didn't come up with the idea first. Remember, your friend or family member would probably love to have you join them but, if you're not interested, that's fine. Just be conscious of your impact on them.

The number one thing you need to do is be aware of those

instinctive, little rebellious thoughts you have when your friend wants to change up his or her routine. It will affect you. Accept that and move on. Your getting irritated because your best friend, mother, or daughter doesn't like to eat at the same places anymore or doesn't like to party like she used to can destroy a health newbie's confidence in a matter of weeks. You must keep in mind that taking control of your health takes some drive, work, commitment, and time.

My program has been designed to drastically limit failure rates associated with diets and fitness programs but, nevertheless, support is still important. In the grand scheme of things, changing up a restaurant or going to a spin class instead of a bar shouldn't matter because what's really important is the time spent together. It's a statistical fact that if your friends tend to be more active and live in a healthier fashion, you will too. Unfortunately, the opposite is true, too. There is a direct correlation between obesity among family members. If a child is overweight or obese, then usually, so are his parents. Furthermore, if a person is heavy, they're also more likely to have heavy friends. Mom was right after all: you are who you hang out with. Why is this? Simple. Our social environment has a profound effect on us. So, supporting a loved one on the Healthy Habit Plan could help you, too. Here are some tips to help your loved one get past the hurdles they're going to meet.

1. **Don't tempt them with bad food.**

    It is the core philosophy of the Healthy Habit Plan that willpower is overrated. In the beginning, it's important to understand that a follower of my program will be riding off limited motivational fuel until habitual patterns start to develop. Eating a deep pan pizza in front of your friend who is desperately trying to change his or her habits is not being supportive—it's being a jerk.

    You have the right to eat and do what you want but so

does someone on my program who is trying to change their eating habits. It's simply a matter of saying, "I'm going to eat this later or in the other room," and then really doing that. Don't give into their plea, "Oh, it's okay." Because it's not, at least not right now. Soon you could open up a fast-food restaurant in your home and it wouldn't tempt them one bit. That's the power of changing your habits. But, until then, it takes time, and they need your help to get there.

2. Don't talk them out of exercise.

Although they are not doing home workouts, coming home after a long day at work and getting geared up for an hour-long spin class takes some motivation, at least to get dressed and get in the car and actually go. Encourage them. Little things like, "I know you're tired but you always feel better after you exercise," or "I'll try to have dinner ready for you" or best of all, "Can I come with you?" does magical things to a person's confidence. Saying things like, "Can't you just work out at home tonight?" or "Please just skip this one night" is selfish because it's really not what they want, it's what *you* want.

Years ago, I trained a woman who really wanted to change her lifestyle and she had this friend who, in my opinion, was the best friend a person could have. The friend hated exercise and had no interest in changing her own lifestyle, but she did something that I thought was so special. She would come with her friend (the woman I was training) to the group training classes and sit on the side and read a book and patiently wait for her friend to finish. She did this for *years.* Pretty soon that overweight woman had become an avid marathon runner who no longer needed my services. I saw her friend a few months back, and she brought me up to date on what she was doing and thanked me for making her best friend so happy. I told her that what I truly believe was one of the main reasons for her friend's success was *her* phenomenal support.

This story is an example of how something as simple as getting in the car and just accompanying a friend to the gym (*and not even doing the workout*) can be powerful enough to make huge differences in a person's life.

3.   Don't be a critic.

The Healthy Habit Plan is a very different program, which sometimes will evoke doubt in those who have been able to achieve health in a different manner. Things like not working out at home, progressive diet approaches, a critical look at supplements, and the doubtful approach to the organic food industry can be seen as a challenge to those whose philosophy to health might differ.

It's important to remember that, like I've said before, the Healthy Habit Plan is not the only road to achieve fitness, but it *is* a very well-paved road and one that is not littered with a high number of fitness casualties.

We are all unique, physically and psychologically. Just because you switched to an all-vegan diet overnight and it worked for you, doesn't mean it will work for your friend. Just because home workouts turned out well for you, doesn't mean they'll work for a loved one. In fact, all you have to do is look at some statistics to realize that, if the above things worked for you, then you are not the norm. You may possess a mental toughness or a strength that your friend doesn't.

Insulting my program or my theories doesn't hurt me; it hurts your friend because they chose the Healthy Habit Plan. It also leads them to start doubting, which usually leads to frustration, which in turn leads to quitting. This is when they may go in search of something that *you* approve of, which may not help them at all because, remember, they are not you. They are their own individual.

So, if you're not a fan of my philosophy, I respect your opinion, but please give me and my program a chance to help your friend. Respect their decision enough to step aside, at least for the time being, and allow them to give it a shot. If it doesn't work, then scoop your friend up in your arms and lead them down your path. But right now, it's my turn.

Bottom line, you have a tremendous amount of influence on your friends and family, and it's a responsibility you shouldn't take lightly. Don't take advantage of your power over them for your own convenience. I believe that, with a little support, you can be the secret weapon that helps your loved ones reach their goals.